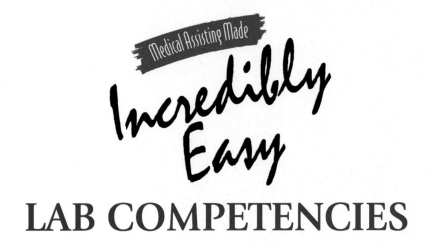

Medical Assisting Made

Incredibly Easy

LAB COMPETENCIES

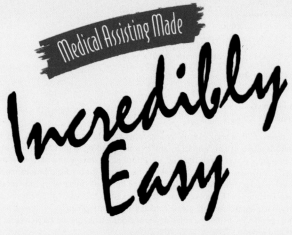

Medical Assisting Made

Incredibly Easy

LAB COMPETENCIES

Peter J. Doolin, MT (ASCP), MEd, RMA

Medical Department
McFatter Technical Center
Davie, Florida

Wolters Kluwer | Lippincott Williams & Wilkins
Health

Philadelphia · Baltimore · New York · London
Buenos Aires · Hong Kong · Sydney · Tokyo

Executive Editor: John Goucher
Senior Managing Editor: Rebecca Kerins
Marketing Manager: Hilary Henderson
Production Editor: Eve Malakoff-Klein
Illustrator: Bot Roda
Designer: Joan Wendt
Compositor: Circle Graphics, Inc.
Printer: R.R. Donnelley & Sons—Crawfordsville

9 8 7 6 5 4 3 2 1

Library of Congress Cataloging-in-Publication Data

Doolin, Peter J.
  Lab competencies / Peter J. Doolin.
    p. ; cm. — (Medical assisting made incredibly easy)
  Includes index.
  ISBN-13: 978-0-7817-6347-9
  ISBN-10: 0-7817-6347-9
  1. Medical assistants. 2. Diagnosis, Laboratory. I. Title. II. Series.
  [DNLM: 1. Clinical Laboratory Techniques—methods—Handbooks. 2. Allied Health Per-
sonnel—Handbooks. QY 25 D691L 2008]
  R728.8.D66 2008
  610.73'7069—dc22

                                    2007001968

DISCLAIMER

Care has been taken to confirm the accuracy of the information present and to describe generally accepted practices. However, the authors, editors, and publisher are not responsible for
errors or omissions or for any consequences from application of the information in this book
and make no warranty, expressed or implied, with respect to the currency, completeness, or accuracy of the contents of the publication. Application of this information in a particular situation
remains the professional responsibility of the practitioner; the clinical treatments described and
recommended may not be considered absolute and universal recommendations.

The authors, editors, and publisher have exerted every effort to ensure that drug selection
and dosage set forth in this text are in accordance with the current recommendations and
practice at the time of publication. However, in view of ongoing research, changes in government regulations, and the constant flow of information relating to drug therapy and drug reactions, the reader is urged to check the package insert for each drug for any change in
indications and dosage and for added warnings and precautions. This is particularly important when the recommended agent is a new or infrequently employed drug.

Some drugs and medical devices presented in this publication have Food and Drug Administration (FDA) clearance for limited use in restricted research settings. It is the responsibility
of the health care provider to ascertain the FDA status of each drug or device planned for use
in their clinical practice.

To purchase additional copies of this book, call our customer service department at **(800) 638-
3030** or fax orders to **(301) 223-2320**. International customers should call **(301) 223-2300**.

Visit Lippincott Williams & Wilkins on the Internet: http://www.lww.com. Lippincott Williams
& Wilkins customer service representatives are available from 8:30 am to 6:00 p.m., EST.

PREFACE

Medical Assisting Made Incredibly Easy is an exciting new series designed to make learning enjoyable for medical assisting students. Each book in the series uses a light-hearted, humorous approach to presenting information. Maria, a Certified Medical Assistant, guides students through the books, offering helpful tips and insights along the way.

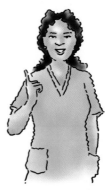

Medical Assisting Made Incredibly Easy takes a practical approach, providing students with the critical information that they need to know, including complete coverage of the core skills they must master in their studies. The series covers all competencies based on the standards and guidelines established for medical assisting by the Commission on Accreditation of Allied Health Educational Programs (CAAHEP) and the Accrediting Bureau of Health Education Schools (ABHES).

ABOUT THIS BOOK

Medical Assisting Made Incredibly Easy: Lab Competencies provides instruction in the clinical competencies related to specimen collection and diagnostic testing covered by CAAHEP and ABHES. These are among the skills that students must master to pass the test required to become either a Certified Medical Assistant or a Registered Medical Assistant.

SPECIAL FEATURES

Medical Assisting Made Incredibly Easy: Lab Competencies is designed to be enjoyable to read, as well as highly informative. Each chapter in this book includes special features designed to guide students in their study. These elements will help students to identify the most important information in the chapter and to understand all of it.

- *Chapter Checklist* includes a list of skills and other important information that students will gain after reading the material.

- **Closer Look** *Closer Look* explores chapter information in more detail in a list or summary form.

- **Running Smoothly** *Running Smoothly* features situations that medical assistants may encounter in a medical office and shows how students can apply what they have learned to those situations.

- **Ask the Professional** *Ask the Professional* offers expert advice on how to handle difficult situations that medical assistants may face in the workplace.

- **Secrets for Success** *Secrets for Success* provides tips for studying, for remembering important material, and for success in a career as a medical assistant.

- **Legal Brief** *Legal Brief* provides important legal and ethical information, including how the Health Insurance Portability and Accountability Act (HIPAA) impacts medical assisting.

- **Word to the Wise** *Word to the Wise* covers terminology that students might find challenging, providing a definition and pronunciation for each term.

- **Your Turn to Teach** *Your Turn To Teach* provides students with valuable information regarding patient education.

- **SAFETY** *Safety First* offers helpful tips and information pertaining to lab safety, an important issue for medical assistants.

- **Hands On** *Hands On* contains procedures for important skills and tasks.

- **Chapter Highlights** *Chapter Highlights* summarizes a chapter's key content.

In addition to the above features, this book also includes bolded key terms throughout each chapter and a Glossary in the back of the book, as well as many other boxed features and tables.

ADDITIONAL RESOURCES

In addition to the text, the following resources are available for students and instructors:

- *Study Guide for Medical Assisting Made Incredibly Easy: Lab Competencies* includes learning activities and exercises, quizzes, puzzles, certification review questions, and competency evaluation forms so students can practice their skills and measure their success.

- An **Online Course** provides interactive exercises and review opportunities that support the text and classroom experience.

- An **Instructor's Resource CD-ROM** with test generator, PowerPoint slides, image bank, answers to study guide questions, and customizable competency evaluation forms helps instructors optimize their teaching. The Instructor's Resource CD-ROM also includes information on where in the book and Study Guide each ABHES and CAAHEP competency is covered.

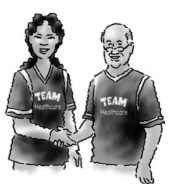

- A complete set of **Lesson Plans** is also available to instructors.

Medical Assisting Made Incredibly Easy: Lab Competencies is designed to make the study of medical assisting fun and effective. The purpose of this book, and the entire *Medical Assisting Made Incredibly Easy* series, is student success!

USER'S GUIDE

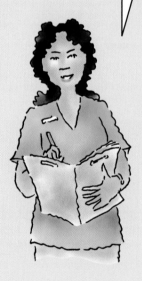

Hello, my name is Maria. I'm a Certified Medical Assistant and educator, as well as your guide through this textbook. There are a number of features in this **Medical Assisting Made Incredibly Easy** text to help you learn everything you need to become a successful medical assistant. Read through this User's Guide to orient yourself to everything the text has to offer. Good luck in your medical assisting studies!

Chapter Checklist

- Explain the purpose of performing clinical chemistry tests
- List the common panels of chemistry tests
- List the instruments used for chemical testing
- List tests used to evaluate renal function
- List the common electrolytes and explain the relationship of electrolytes to body function
- Describe the nonprotein nitrogenous compounds and name conditions associated with abnormal values
- Describe the substances commonly tested in liver function assessment
- Explain thyroid function and identify the hormone that regulates the thyroid gland
- Describe how laboratory tests help assess for a myocardial infarction
- Describe how pancreatitis is diagnosed with laboratory tests
- Explain how the body uses and regulates glucose and summarize the purpose of the major glucose tests
- Determine a patient's blood glucose level
- Perform glucose tolerance testing
- Describe the function of cholesterol and other lipids and their correlation to heart disease

Chapter Checklists orient you to the material that's covered in the current chapter.

Closer Look — THE QUALITY CONTROL LOG

A lab must keep a QC log to show compliance with CLIA testing requirements. The log can be kept as a book or on the computer. It must include a record of each control sample and standard test. Here's what these entries must contain:

- the date and time of the test
- the results expected
- the results obtained
- the action taken for correction, if necessary

Your office m[...]
on maintenan[...]
kept in the Q[...]

Closer Look boxes explore topics in more detail.

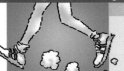

Running Smoothly — PACKAGING SPECIMENS FOR REFERENCE LABS

How can I protect the specimens I send to a reference lab?

Specimens sent to off-site labs have to be packaged carefully to prevent damage that can occur from:

- rough handling
- very high or low temperatures
- pressure changes

Containers that meet federal regulations for transporting biohazardous materials must be used. These containers are designed to protect the specimens and are leak proof.

Running Smoothly boxes feature situations that you may encounter in a medical office and teach you to apply what you've learned to those situations.

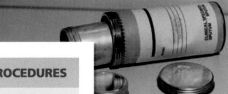

[...]d specimens to a lab protect both the contents

Ask the Professional — FOLLOWING BLOOD DRAW PROCEDURES

Q: *I've noticed that one of my coworkers is not following the proper procedures for blood draw. I feel like I should say something, but we are friends outside of work. I want to keep our friendship. What should I do?*

A: Yes, you should talk with your coworker. It may be uncomfortable for you, but remember that you're a medical professional and you must act like one. You have a legal and ethical responsibility to make sure patients get the best possible care. Talk to your friend at a time when both of you are relaxed. Tell her that you've noticed she's not following the blood draw procedure you learned and that you'd like to help. Be willing to listen to her side of the situation and give her the benefit of the doubt. She may be unsure of the proper procedures to follow.

If you find that your coworker has not corrected the problem after you have talked, then you should talk to your supervisor.

Ask the Professional boxes offer expert advice on how to handle difficult situations that you may face in the workplace.

Secrets for Success boxes provide tips for studying, for remembering important material, and for success in your career as a medical assistant.

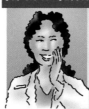

Secrets for Success   **WORKING THE SYRINGE PLUNGER**

When you try to pull the plunger on a new syringe, the plunger may stick at first. This happens because the lubricant on the plunger forms a seal inside the barrel that must be broken for the plunger to move freely. You can make the plunger easier to move by using a technique called breathing the syringe. Before inserting the needle, pull back the plunger to about halfway up the barrel. Then push it back. Now the plunger will move more smoothly.

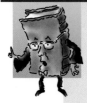

Legal Brief   **TEST RESULTS AND PATIENT PRIVACY**

As a medical assistant, you'll have access to sensitive test results, such as those for:

• human immunodeficiency virus (HIV)
• pregnancy
• illegal drugs
• sexually transmitted diseases (STDs)

You have a responsibility to keep the results of these tests, *or any test results*, from unauthorized persons. Only the physician and the patient are entitled to the results. The only exception is when laws require reporting certain results to protect public health and safety. However, deciding when

Legal Briefs provide important legal and ethical information, including how the Health Insurance Portability and Accountability Act (HIPAA) affects your work in the medical office.

Word to the Wise   **centrifugal force** (sen-TRIF-uh guhl FORS)

a spinning motion to exert force outward; heavier components of a solution are spun downward

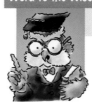

Word to the Wise boxes cover terminology that you might find challenging, providing a definition and pronunciation for each term.

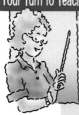

Your Turn to Teach   **COLLECTING SPECIMENS FROM PATIENTS**

Before collecting a patient's specimen, you should provide the patient with the following information:

• the name of the test (such as a blood cell count test)
• the type of specimen the patient will give (such as blood, urine, or stool)
• what kind of preparation the patient needs to do (such as fasting or following a certain diet)
• the purpose of the test
• how long it will take to get results back from the lab
• how the patient will be told the results

Proper preparation is especially important. In testing for diabetes for example, if the patient doesn't prepare properly, the test results may be wrong.

Your Turn To Teach boxes provide helpful information about patient education.

Safety First boxes offer tips and information about lab safety, an important issue for medical assistants.

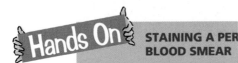

MATERIAL SAFETY DATA SHEETS

An MSDS is required for each hazardous material at your workplace. Many of the chemicals used for lab tests are hazardous. But so are many materials used for everyday office maintenance. They can include disinfectants, cleaning compounds, and even office supplies like printer toner! They all must be labeled as hazardous with the contents listed on the label.

Hands On — STAINING A PER BLOOD SMEAR

To stain a peripheral blood smear, you'll need the following equipment: a staining rack, Wright's stain, Giemsa stain, a prepared slide, and tweezers.

Follow these steps to stain a peripheral blood smear:

1. Wash your hands.
2. Get your equipment ready.
3. Put on gloves, an impervious gown, and a face shield.
4. Get the dried blood smear. Keep in mind that a smear made from blood that's more that four hours old may have deteriorated cells.
5. Place the slide on a stain rack, blood side up. Then, flood the slide with Wright's stain. Leave the stain on the slide for three to five minutes or for the time specified by the manufacturer. The alcohol in Wright's stain helps fix the blood to the slide.
6. Use your tweezers to tilt the slide so that the stain drains off. Then, apply equal amounts of Giemsa stain and water or a Wright's buffer. A green sheen will appear on the slide's surface. Let the solution remain on the slide for five minutes or the time specified by the manufacturer. This helps improve the quality of the stain.
7. Again, hold the slide with your tweezers. Gently rinse the slide with water to remove any excess stain. Wipe off the back of the slide with gauze. Stand the slide upright and allow it to dry.
8. Properly take care of or dispose of equipment and supplies. Clean your work a
   face shield, and w:

Note: Some manufac
sists of dipping the sr
and then rinsing. Dir
with the specific stain

Hands On boxes contain step-by-step, easy-to-follow procedures for important skills and tasks.

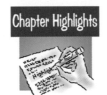 Chapter Highlights

- A blood drawing station has the supplies and equipment needed for phlebotomy procedures.
- The venipuncture systems are the evacuated tube system and the syringe system.
- Venipuncture uses color-coded stoppers to identify the additive content of each type of tube.
- Blood specimens collected by venipuncture must be placed in evacuated tubes in proper order of draw.
- Lancets are used to pierce the skin to collect drops of blood in skin puncture.
- It's essential to identify the patient before performing a venipuncture or skin puncture.
- Hematoma is the most common complication of venipuncture.

Chapter Highlights summarize a chapter's key content.

REVIEWERS

Julie Akason, BSN, MAEd
College of St. Catherine
St. Paul, Minnesota

Nina Beaman, MS, BA, AAS
Bryant and Stratton College
Richmond, Virginia

Mary-Elizabeth Browder, BA, CMA, MEd
Raymond Walters College
Cincinnati, Ohio

Michelle Carfagna, BS
Brevard Community College
Cocoa, Florida

Tracie Fuqua, BS
Wallace State Community College
Hanceville, Alabama

Rebecca Gibson-Lee, MSTE, CMA, ASPT
The University of Akron
Akron, Ohio

Robyn Gohsman, AAS
Medical Careers Institute
Newport News, Virginia

Christine Golden, MS, MT (ASCP)
Waukesha County Technical College
Pewaukee, Wisconsin

Rebecca Hickey, RN, RMC, AHI, CHI, BA
Butler Technology and Career
Development Schools
Fairfield Township, Ohio

Joanna Holly, RN, BS, MS
Midstate College
Peoria, Illinois

Dorothy Kiel, BS
Rhodes State College
Lima, Ohio

Carol Lacy, RN, BSN, PHN
College of Marin
Novato, California

Maureen Messier, AS, BA
Branford Hall Career Institute
Southington, Connecticut

Lisa Nagle, BSEd, CMA
Augusta Technical College
Augusta, Georgia

Eva Oltman, MAEd
Jefferson Community and Technical College
Louisville, Kentucky

Cheryl Startzell, MA, BS, AAS
San Antonio College
San Antonio, Texas

Kathy Steinberg, RN, BSN
Midwest Technical Institute
Lincoln, Illinois

Nina Thierer, BS
Ivy Tech Community College
Fort Wayne, Indiana

Stacey Wilson, BS, MT/PBT, CMA
Cabarrus College of Health Sciences
Concord, North Carolina

CONTENTS

PREFACE   v

USER'S GUIDE   ix

REVIEWERS   xiii

Chapter 1
GETTING TO KNOW THE CLINICAL LAB   1

Chapter 2
PHLEBOTOMY   35

Chapter 3
HEMATOLOGY   74

Chapter 4
IMMUNOLOGY AND IMMUNOHEMATOLOGY   110

Chapter 5
URINALYSIS   136

Chapter 6
CLINICAL CHEMISTRY   181

Chapter 7
MICROBIOLOGY   214

GLOSSARY   275

FIGURE CREDITS   285

INDEX   287

GETTING TO KNOW THE CLINICAL LAB

Chapter Checklist

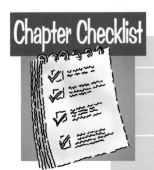

- List the reasons for lab tests

- Describe the medical assistant's role in the lab

- Identify the kinds of labs where medical assistants work and describe what these labs do

- List the kinds of people who work in a lab and the duties of each

- Name each type of lab department and explain what it does

- List the equipment found in most small labs and explain its purpose

- Identify the kinds of hazards encountered in a lab and summarize how to deal with them

- Explain how OSHA makes labs safer

- List the safe behaviors employees should practice in the lab

- Identify CLIA and explain how it affects lab operations

- Describe how quality control affects lab operations

Laboratories test a person's blood, urine, and other body samples to help identify diseases and disorders. In this chapter, you will learn about the different types of laboratories where a medical assistant might work. You'll also learn how to use a microscope and other tools, as well as about safety on the job.

Labs and What They Do

Lab results are compared with what are called **normal values.** Normal values are acceptable ranges for healthy people. Lab results can be used to assess the health of a particular organ or to tell if a patient's medication dosage is correct.

The most common laboratory testing is used to:

- diagnose disease
- determine the progress of a disease or its response to treatment
- perform legal blood tests, such as for drug testing or a marriage license

Some other common tests might be used to:

- monitor a patient's medication and treatment
- find the levels of key substances in the body
- find out the cause of an infection
- determine a baseline value
- prevent disease

LABORATORIES AND YOU

As a medical assistant, you'll have responsibilities of many kinds to both your patients and your doctor. Your role in lab testing will be vital because such tests provide some of the most powerful diagnostic tools there are.

You'll need to tell patients how to collect their own **specimens,** or samples, such as stool or urine. This is to be sure they provide quality specimens—those that are free from contamination.

Some of the more common lab tests are ones you may be asked to do right in the office where you work. At other times, you'll need to arrange for sending the specimens to the lab if it is off-site.

One of the most important duties you'll have is keeping records through a **quality assurance (QA)** program. Among other things, QA helps ensure good patient care. A good QA program includes **quality control (QC)** processes. These help ensure accuracy in testing by monitoring things like:

- supplies and instruments
- policies and procedures
- equipment

You also may be in charge of buying lab supplies and choosing **reagents,** or the chemicals used to produce a test reaction.

Biohazard safety and waste disposal are two critical areas you may be responsible for as well.

TYPES OF LABS

The three types of labs you may deal with are reference labs, hospital labs, and physician office labs (POLs).

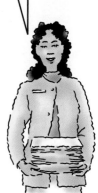

Reference and hospital labs process and report on thousands of specimens each day.

- Reference and hospital labs do hundreds of specialized tests each day.
- POLs perform only a few types of tests on a limited number of patients.

Reference Laboratories

A reference lab is sometimes called a *referral laboratory*. It is large and much like a factory. Many tests are done there each day. A reference lab gets specimens from many different places, such as doctors' offices, hospitals, and clinics. This kind of lab rarely sees patients directly.

Tests at a reference lab are done in bulk "runs." Specimens from many patients are tested at the same time. The results are put into a computer and reported to the patients' doctors. Each physician then gives the results to the patient.

Specimens sent to a reference lab can be delivered by these methods:

- special courier
- U.S. mail
- ground delivery service
- air delivery service

Hospital Laboratories

A hospital lab serves patients who are in the hospital for both long and short stays. The hospital lab staff includes:

- **phlebotomists** (fleb-AH-tuh-mists), who draw blood from patients
- lab assistants, who collect and process specimens
- lab technicians and medical technologists, who perform most of the testing
- secretaries or receptionists, who process patients and manage the lab's paperwork.

What would your role be in all of this? You might act as a secretary or receptionist, a lab assistant, or even a phlebotomist. It all depends upon your job description.

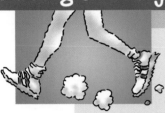

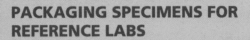

Running Smoothly

PACKAGING SPECIMENS FOR REFERENCE LABS

How can I protect the specimens I send to a reference lab?

Specimens sent to off-site labs have to be packaged carefully to prevent damage that can occur from:

- rough handling
- very high or low temperatures
- pressure changes

Containers that meet federal regulations for transporting biohazardous materials must be used. These containers are designed to protect the specimens and are leak proof.

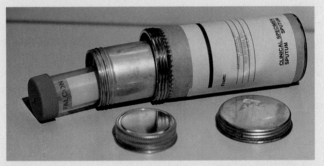

The special containers used to send specimens to a lab protect both the contents and those who handle the package.

The most common tests in hospitals are performed right there. More specialized tests may be sent to a reference lab for processing. But no matter which of these labs does the testing, the results are usually ready in 24 to 48 hours.

Physician Office Labs

The most common type of lab is the POL, or physician office laboratory. Most POLs only do low-difficulty tests. However, some more difficult tests may sometimes be done in a POL too.

The most common tests done in a POL include:

- urinalysis
- blood cell counts
- hemoglobin and hematocrit

- blood glucose
- cholesterol levels

Pregnancy tests and quick screening tests, such as for mononucleosis or strep throat, also may be done in a POL.

If you're working in a POL, you could be responsible for (under physician supervision):

- collecting samples
- performing tests
- managing QC
- maintaining lab instruments
- keeping records
- reporting results

LAB DEPARTMENTS

POLs may have only one department. But larger labs do so many tests that they need special departments to handle all the types. Here are the basic departments usually found in a hospital or reference lab.

- hematology department
- clinical chemistry department
- immunology department

Your Turn to Teach

COLLECTING SPECIMENS FROM PATIENTS

Before collecting a patient's specimen, you should provide the patient with the following information:

- the name of the test (such as a blood cell count test)
- the type of specimen the patient will give (such as blood, urine, or stool)
- the purpose of the test
- what kind of preparation the patient needs to do (such as fasting or following a certain diet)
- how long it will take to get results back from the lab
- how the patient will be told the results

Proper preparation is especially important. In testing for diabetes for example, if the patient doesn't prepare properly, the test results may be wrong.

- microbiology department
- pathology department
- immunohematology department (also known as the "blood bank")

Hematology

The hematology department tests for various types of cells in the blood and how many of each type are present. Common tests include:

- complete blood count (CBC)
- white blood cell count (WBC)
- platelet count
- hemoglobin and hematocrit (H & H)
- differential
- erythrocyte sedimentary rate (ESR or "sed rate")
- reticulocyte count

Coagulation is also often part of the hematology department. These tests tell how well the body responds when blood vessels are damaged. The most common tests are:

- prothrombin time (PT)
- partial prothrombin time (PPT)
- fibrogen
- bleeding time

These tests are also used to check levels of **anticoagulant** medicines, such as heparin and Coumadin. Anticoagulant medicines prevent blood clotting in conditions caused by clot formation and blocked blood vessels. These conditions include heart attacks, strokes, pulmonary embolisms, some types of phlebitis, and others.

Clinical Chemistry

The clinical chemistry department measures chemical substances in the blood. Examples include:

- hormones and enzymes
- medicines and drugs
- sugars, proteins, and fats
- waste products

The most common chemistry tests performed in a small lab are:

- glucose
- cholesterol

- blood urea nitrogen (BUN)
- electrolytes

Toxicology is often a separate part of a chemistry department. Toxicology testing involves measuring levels of both medical drugs and illegal drugs in a person's blood.

Immunohematology

The immunohematology department is commonly known as the blood bank. This department is found only in hospitals and blood donor centers. It does blood typing and makes sure a stored blood product can be given safely to a patient who needs a transfusion.

Immunology

Immunology is sometimes called serology. This department tests for certain diseases based on the reactions of antibodies to foreign substances in the body. Immunology tests are used to detect HIV, mononucleosis, syphilis, and other diseases.

Microbiology

The microbiology department identifies **microorganisms** that cause disease and which drugs will combat them most effectively. Microorganisms are living organisms that can only be seen with the aid of a microscope. The specialties within the microbiology department include:

- bacteriology, or the study of bacteria
- virology, or the study of viruses

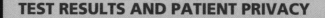

Legal Brief　　TEST RESULTS AND PATIENT PRIVACY

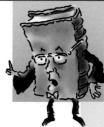

As a medical assistant, you'll have access to sensitive test results, such as those for:

- human immunodeficiency virus (HIV)
- pregnancy
- illegal drugs
- sexually transmitted diseases (STDs)

You have a responsibility to keep the results of these tests, *or any test results*, from unauthorized persons. Only the physician and the patient are entitled to the results. The only exception is when laws require reporting certain results to protect public health and safety. However, deciding when to do this won't be your responsibility.

Closer Look   URINALYSIS

The urinalysis department is often part of another department. It can be included in the chemistry, hematology, or microbiology department. Urinalysis looks at the physical, chemical, and microscopic properties of urine. Pregnancy tests often are done in this department.

- mycology, or the study of fungi and yeasts
- parasitology, or the study of parasites (for example, certain protozoa and worms)

Anatomical and Surgical Pathology

The pathology department studies specimens from:

- aspirations—fluids or gases suctioned from a body cavity
- biopsies—living tissue surgically removed for examination
- autopsies—examinations of dead bodies
- surgically removed organs

Pathology departments usually have histology and cytology sections. In larger labs, however, histology and cytology may be departments of their own.

Histology is the study of tissue. Tissue samples are prepared and studied under a microscope to show if disease is present. Biopsies and frozen specimens that need immediate results are often examined in this department.

Cytology is the study of cells. Individual cells in body fluids and other types of specimens are studied under a microscope to find things like cancer or other disease. The most common cytology test is the Papanicolaou (Pap) test in which cells from a woman's cervix are evaluated.

Cytogenetics is a special form of cytology that examines the genetic information contained in cells for data. Cells can be obtained from tissue, blood, or other body fluids. They are examined for DNA deficiencies related to disease.

WHO WORKS IN A LAB?

The various lab departments employ many people to carry out their duties. Most jobs require specific education or training. The table on page 9 summarizes the kinds of people who work in labs.

Typical Lab Employees

Who They Are	What They Do
Pathologist	A pathologist is a doctor who studies disease. Usually, a pathologist manages the technical parts of a lab.
Chief technologist or lab manager	This person supervises the lab. The chief technologist manages the day-to-day events, including: • staffing • pricing • purchasing • quality control • the test "menu"
Certified medical technologist	A certified medical technologist is specially trained in a four-year college program and nationally certified. This individual performs all levels of lab tests according to CLIA rules.
Medical laboratory technician	A medical laboratory technician has completed one year of college and one year of clinical training. This person performs lab tests but is not in a supervising position.
Medical assistant	This individual is a high school graduate or equivalent who has completed a medical assistant program at a community college or technical school. A medical assistant may collect and process specimens and perform waived laboratory procedures.
Laboratory assistant	A laboratory assistant is a high school graduate or equivalent who has completed a vocational or on-the-job training program. This person collects and processes specimens and may perform some tests.
Phlebotomist	This individual is trained to draw blood and process specimens. Phlebotomists can have additional duties that are more involved. Sometimes they are also medical or laboratory assistants.
Histologist	A histologist is trained to process and evaluate tissue samples, such as biopsies.
Cytologist	A cytologist is a professional trained to look for abnormal changes in cells under a microscope.
Specimen processor or accessioner	A specimen processor is trained to accept shipments of specimens and to prepare them for testing. This individual labels and numbers the specimens and enters the specimen data into a computer.

PHYSICIAN OFFICE LAB TESTING

The federal government regulates the kinds of tests that can be performed by a physician office lab. In general, only two kinds of tests can be conducted in a POL.

• tests done on semi-automated machines

• tests done with self-contained test kits

The instructions in test kits are the best source of information on how to conduct those tests safely and accurately.

So are the instructions inside packages of reagents for test machines and QC instructions for the machines themselves. Information from these sources should be combined with the POL's routine procedures to provide written instructions for each test it performs.

Legal Brief   CHAIN OF CUSTODY

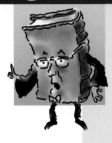

When you work in a lab, you may be in charge of collecting specimens for drug or other testing done for legal purposes. A chain of custody (COC) is a process that accounts for a specimen at all times. A COC form is signed by each person who handles the specimen until the testing is complete. This procedure documents that the specimen is genuine and that no one has tampered with it.

For example, here are some basic requirements for testing a subject's urine for illegal drugs.

- Obtain a picture ID and have the subject empty his pockets before collecting the specimen.
- The water supply in the restroom used for collection must be turned off. A dye must be added to toilet water to prevent the subject from using it as the specimen.
- Record whether or not collection of the specimen was witnessed.
- Record the specimen's temperature (90.5 to 99.8 degrees F is acceptable). Its minimum volume should be 35 mL.
- Have the subject and the collector sign the COC form, with the date and time of collection.
- Sign and attach tamper seals to each side of the container, going across the lid.
- Put the specimen and COC form in a tamper-proof bag.
- Seal the bag for transport to the testing facility.

LABORATORY EQUIPMENT

There are many types of lab equipment, but you only need to know a few of them well. Here are the types of basic equipment with which you should be familiar:

- microscope
- centrifuge

- chemistry analyzer
- incubator
- glassware
- lab refrigerator or freezer
- automated cell counter

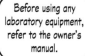
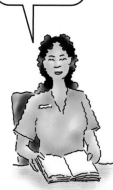

Before using any laboratory equipment, refer to the owner's manual.

Microscopes

A microscope is used to identify cells and microorganisms (sometimes called **microbes**) in specimens. The microscope most commonly used in a POL is a compound microscope. It has two lenses to magnify the object you're observing. A strong light helps you see the object better.

Here are the basic parts of a compound microscope.

- The *frame* is the main part of the microscope. It holds the *arm* and the *base*.
- The *eyepiece* or *ocular* at the top of the microscope is what you look through. Binocular microscopes have two eyepieces. This causes less eyestrain.
- The *adjustment knobs* are used to bring the object you're looking at into focus.
- The *stage* is the flat surface that holds the slide you are studying. The stage has clips or guides to control the slide's movement.
- The *condenser* focuses the light onto the slide. The lower the position of the condenser, the less light you will have. The higher the position, the brighter the light will be.
- The *diaphragm* is part of the condenser. It acts like the iris in your eye, in that its opening can be adjusted to allow for more or less light. The more highly magnified the slide is, the greater the need for light.
- The *light source* is housed in the microscope's base.

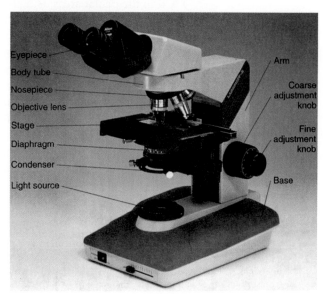

Basic components of the standard light microscope. (Courtesy of Nikon, Melville, NY.)
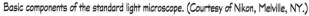

MICROSCOPE STORAGE

Microscopes are delicate and expensive instruments. They must be handled and stored properly to stay in good working order. Here are some rules to follow when storing a microscope.

- Make sure the light source is turned off and rotate the nosepiece until the lowest-power lens faces the stage.
- Cover the microscope when it's not being used.
- Be sure to keep it in a place where there isn't a lot of traffic.
- Make sure it's away from any source of vibration, such as a **centrifuge**.

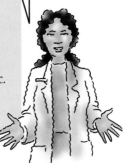

Be careful when lifting a microscope. It's a lot heavier than it looks!

Closer Look

CARING FOR A MICROSCOPE

Here are some tips for cleaning the microscope in your lab.

- As with any lab procedure, wash your hands before getting started.
- Assemble the equipment and use both hands to carry the microscope. You should use one hand on the base and the other on the arm of the microscope.
- Clean the ocular areas using lens paper and cleaner. Don't use gauze or tissue, as these may scratch the glass. Don't touch the glass with your fingers.
- Start with the eyepiece—or ocular—and work down to the lenses near the base. Clean each piece of glass. Change lens paper often, once you see it's getting dirty. The cleanest area of a microscope is usually the eyepiece and the dirtiest is the highest-power lens.
- Use a clean lens paper to wipe each ocular area *again* to make sure no dirt and cleaner is left behind. If there is, whatever you're examining under the microscope can look distorted.
- All other areas of the microscope (like the stage, the base, and the knobs) can be cleaned using a mild soap solution and gauze. These should be cleaned regularly to keep oil and dirt from building up.
- Cover the microscope at the end of the day.

Centrifuge

A centrifuge is a machine that separates liquids into their different parts. It does this by using centrifugal force, or spinning that exerts force outward. The heavier parts of the liquid are pushed farther out from the center than the lighter parts are. This action separates the liquid.

Here's what happens when a blood specimen is spun in a centrifuge.

- The heavier part of the blood goes to the bottom of the tube. This part of the blood is made up of red blood cells.
- A middle layer, known as the **buffy coat,** forms. This contains the specimen's WBC and platelets.
- The topmost layer of separated blood can have two different names. It's known as **plasma** if the specimen was from an anticoagulated tube (lavender, blue, gray, or yellow tube tops). If the specimen was allowed to clot (in a red tube top), its top layer is called **serum.** Serum and plasma are straw colored and look identical. However, there are chemical differences.

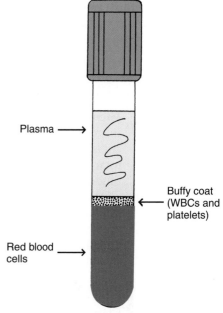

Plasma

Buffy coat (WBCs and platelets)

Red blood cells

Here is an example of a centrifuged blood specimen.

Working with a Centrifuge. Here are some facts you should know before working with a centrifuge.

- Tubes spun in a centrifuge always must be in an even number and balanced. An unbalanced centrifuge may "walk" along the table and fall off the top.

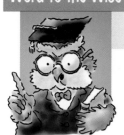

Word to the Wise

centrifugal force (sen-TRIF-uh guhl FORS)

a spinning motion to exert force outward; heavier components of a solution are spun downward

- The tubes all should have about the same level of liquid and they should be tightly capped.
- Never run the centrifuge until you've locked the lid.
- Wait until the centrifuge has stopped spinning before opening it.
- Don't use your hand to try and stop the spinning—this could be dangerous.
- The centrifuge must be cleaned, oiled, and maintained regularly. Follow the manufacturer's instructions as to how to do this.

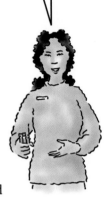

Here's a tip to use when your centrifuge holds four tubes, but you have only three tubes to spin. Fill a tube with water and use it as the fourth tube to keep the centrifuge balanced.

Microhematocrit. A special type of centrifuge called a microhematocrit is used to run a hematocrit test. The hematocrit is the amount of packed red blood cells compared to the total volume of the sample. This test tells the percentage of red blood cells in whole blood.

The hematocrit test requires a special test tube called a capillary tube. This is a very small tube used for collecting and testing tiny blood samples. One end of the tube is sealed with clay and placed in the centrifuge with this end to the outside. Then the tube is spun.

Chemistry Analyzers

Chemistry analyzers are machines used for doing multiple tests on a sample. Complex analyzers can perform 30 or more tests and are operated by computer.

Some analyzers are handheld and can be moved easily. They're simple to use and don't require a large sample. Best of all, they can give results within minutes. A computer shows the results on the screen or it can give a printout of the results.

POLs use bench-top analyzers when they conduct a variety of chemistry tests or do a lot of testing. Some of these machines use wet reagent systems. A separate reagent pack is required for each type of test.

Other chemistry analyzers use dry reagent technology. All the test reagents are put on a special strip or card, which is put into the machine. Then a drop of blood or serum is added to the strip with a special pipet. (You will read about pipets next.)

Glassware

Glassware includes glass and—believe it or not—plastic too. Plastic is great because it's not as breakable as glass and it's disposable once it has been contaminated. Here are some examples of the glassware you might use in the lab.

Beaker. A beaker is a container with a wide opening for mixing or heating liquids.

Flask. A flask is a container with a narrow opening and round base for holding or moving liquids. There are many different kinds of flasks.

Glass Slides. Glass slides and coverslips are used to hold a specimen for viewing under a microscope. Because they get contaminated by the specimen, these are usually disposable.

Graduated Cylinder. A graduated cylinder is a container used for measuring liquids. **Graduated** means it's marked with divisions—usually in milliliters (mL) for exact measurements.

Petri Dish or Plate. A petri dish or plate is a shallow covered dish filled with a substance that grows the microbes in a specimen.

Pipet or Pipette. A pipet or pipette is used to move or measure small amounts of liquid. Manual pipets have mostly been replaced by mechanical ones. Mechanical pipets come in either fixed or variable sizes and have replaceable tips. They're easier to use and care for than the old manual pipets.

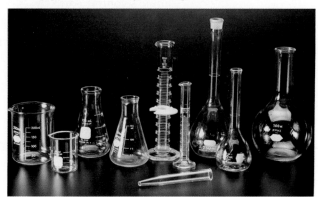

Test Tube. A test tube is a straw-shaped container that's open at one end and round or pointed at the other. It's used to hold lab specimens.

Here's a variety of beakers, flasks, graduated cylinders, and a test tube.

Other Lab Equipment

Here's other equipment commonly found in a lab with which you also should be familiar.

Incubator. An *incubator* is used to keep microbiology specimens at a certain temperature (usually about 95 to 99 degrees F or 35 to 37 degrees C). You'll notice that this is close to body temperature. Some bacteria and other microbes must be this warm to grow and reproduce. Lab employees should keep a daily log that records the incubator's temperature.

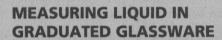

Closer Look

MEASURING LIQUID IN GRADUATED GLASSWARE

The surface of liquid in a glass container isn't flat. It's curved instead. That's because the glass attracts the liquid, which pulls it up the container's sides. The curved surface of the liquid that results is called the meniscus. The narrower the container, the more curved the meniscus will be.

- Measure liquid in graduated glassware by where the *bottom* of the meniscus is located, not at its edges.

- When measuring to obtain a specific volume of liquid, place enough into the container to bring the meniscus above the line for the amount desired (drawing A).

- Remove liquid using a Pasteur pipette with a bulb until the bottom of the meniscus touches the desired graduation line (drawing B).

- The illustrations show this process and how to read a liquid's volume correctly.

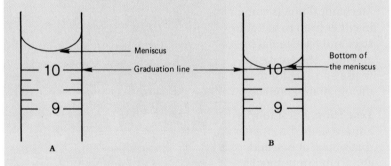

Refrigerators and Freezers. *Refrigerators* and *freezers* in the lab may look like yours at home, but they may be very different. They're used to store reagents, kits, and specimens. Like the incubator, keeping the temperature constant is vital. The temperature should be recorded daily.

Automated Cell Counter. An *automated cell counter* tests blood specimens for white and red blood cell counts plus hematocrit and hemoglobin levels. Some might be used for platelet counts as well. Many counters perform calculations (called indices) and a basic WBC differential. Using a cell counter requires special training from a qualified person.

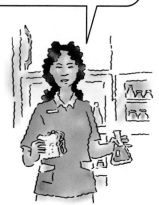

Storing food in a lab refrigerator is a danger to your health and violates OSHA regulations. Specimens contain diseases that could be transferred to your food!

Lab Safety

People who work in a lab must pay special attention to safety. Every specimen should be treated as if it's hazardous. To avoid injury to yourself or others, you also should be aware of the three basic types of hazards in a lab.

- physical hazards
- chemical hazards
- biological hazards

Everyone in your workplace should be aware of how to handle each type of hazard. There should be written policies and procedures designed to keep risks to a minimum.

PHYSICAL HAZARDS

Physical hazards include fires, broken glass, or spills that could cause someone to slip and fall.

If a fire breaks out, all employees should know where the fire extinguishers are located. You also must know how to use one. It's equally important to know all the escape routes out of the lab.

With so much equipment in the average lab, the risk from electrical fires is especially high. Follow these precautions to help avoid electrical fires.

- Don't use extension cords.
- Don't overload electrical outlets.
- Unplug equipment before servicing or repairing it.

CHEMICAL HAZARDS

Chemical hazards involve substances that create fumes or could hurt you by coming into contact with your eyes or skin. Other chemical hazards arise from chemicals that could catch fire or explode.

All chemicals should come with a **material safety data sheet (MSDS)**. Each chemical's MSDS gives the manufacturer's instructions for how to store, handle, and dispose of it. The MSDS also contains information about:

- the chemical's risks
- how to prevent exposure to it
- how to treat exposure to it

All MSDSs should be kept in a binder in the lab. This lets you look up the safety procedures for each chemical easily. The binder also should contain the lab's own rules and procedures for handling hazardous chemicals.

To reduce chemical hazards, read each bottle's label for storage information. Failure to read this storage information can result in:

- damage to the chemical
- release of fumes that could be dangerous and should have been vented
- improper placement of two chemicals next to each other that could result in a reaction between the two stored reagents

BIOLOGICAL HAZARDS

Your lab's binder should include rules and procedures for the handling of test specimens as well. Nearly all types of specimens are capable of passing on disease if they contain microbes that cause the disease. Most of the biological hazards in a lab relate to possible exposure to these microbes.

Lab accidents and careless procedures could result in dangerous exposures. Some of the worst are exposure to the microbes that cause diseases such as:

 MATERIAL SAFETY DATA SHEETS

An MSDS is required for each hazardous material at your workplace. Many of the chemicals used for lab tests are hazardous. But so are many materials used for everyday office maintenance. They can include disinfectants, cleaning compounds, and even office supplies like printer toner! They all must be labeled as hazardous with the contents listed on the label.

- HIV/AIDS
- hepatitis
- tuberculosis

In some cases, you may be testing for such diseases. At other times, you'll be handling specimens from patients that have infectious diseases, although no one may suspect it.

To reduce the risks from biological hazards, the Occupational Safety and Health Administration (OSHA) requires you to wear personal protective equipment (PPE) in the lab. You will read more about OSHA requirements shortly.

THE NATIONAL FIRE PROTECTION ASSOCIATION HAZARDOUS MATERIALS RATING

The National Fire Protection Association (NFPA) has a labeling system to identify the risks from various hazardous chemicals. This system uses a diamond-shaped symbol divided into four sections, each with a different color.

- Blue means health hazard.
- Red means fire hazard.
- Yellow means reactive hazard, such as an explosion.
- White is left blank unless there's a specific hazard, such as radiation, or a reaction if a substance comes into contact with water.

A number from zero (little or no danger) to four (great danger) appears in each color section. This number rates the seriousness of that type of hazard. The ratings will depend on what chemicals are used and stored in the area.

Hazardous materials posters should be displayed in all lab areas, in places where they're easy to see. You should know the NFPA system well enough to understand what each poster means. The illustration on page 20 will tell you more about the system.

OCCUPATIONAL SAFETY AND HEALTH ADMINISTRATION REQUIREMENTS

The Occupational Safety and Health Administration (OSHA) is a federal government agency that protects the health and safety of all workers. OSHA standards are designed to reduce, eliminate, or prevent hazards and accidents in the workplace. OSHA requirements must be followed, even if they conflict with the regulations of other agencies.

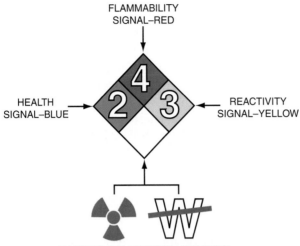

RADIOACTIVE OR WATER REACTIVE

Identification of Health Hazard Color Code: **BLUE**		Identification of Flammability Color Code: **RED**		Identification of Reactivity (Stability) Color Code: **YELLOW**	
	Type of possible injury		Susceptibility of materials to burning		Susceptibility to release of energy
SIGNAL		SIGNAL		SIGNAL	
4	Materials that on very short exposure could cause death or major residual injury even though prompt medical treatment was given.	4	Materials that will rapidly or completely vaporize at atmospheric pressure and normal ambient temperature, or that are readily dispersed in air and that will burn readily.	4	Materials that in themselves are readily capable of detonation or of explosive decomposition or reaction at normal temperatures and pressures.
3	Materials that on short exposure could cause serious temporary or residual injury even though prompt medical treatment was given.	3	Liquids and solids that can be ignited under almost all ambient temperature conditions.	3	Materials that in themselves are capable of detonation or explosive reaction but require a strong initiating source or that must be heated under confinement before initiation or that react explosively with water.
2	Materials that on intense or continued exposure could cause temporary incapacitation or possible residual injury unless prompt medical treatment is given.	2	Materials that must be moderately heated or exposed to relatively high ambient temperatures before ignition can occur.	2	Materials that in themselves are normally unstable and readily undergo violent chemical change but do not detonate. Also materials that may react violently with water or that may form potentially explosive mixtures with water.
1	Materials that on exposure would cause irritation but only minor residual injury even if no treatment is given.	1	Materials that must be preheated before ignition can occur.	1	Materials that in themselves are normally stable, but that can become unstable at elevated temperatures and pressures or that may react with water with some release of energy, but not violently.
0	Materials that on exposure under fire conditions would offer no hazard beyond that of ordinary combustible material.	0	Materials that will not burn.	0	Materials that in themselves are normally stable, even under fire exposure conditions, and that are not reactive with water.

Here's the NFPA hazardous materials rating system.

Two very important OSHA standards that apply to medical labs are:

- the Occupational Exposure to Bloodborne Pathogens Standard
- the Hazardous Communication (HazCom) Standard

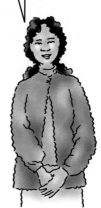

The Hazardous Communication Standard is also known as the "right to know" law.

Bloodborne Pathogens Standard

OSHA requires that all lab personnel be trained to protect themselves from contact with **bloodborne pathogens.** These are dangerous organisms than can exist in the blood of an infected person. The standard also applies to all other body fluids and secretions.

Lab duties carry the risk of exposure to such pathogens. If you're punctured accidentally by a needle or if any body fluid splashes into your eyes, nose, mouth, or other opening in your skin, you could be at risk.

One of the most vital protections your employer must provide is free immunization for you against hepatitis B virus and other bloodborne pathogens. This must happen within ten days of your being assigned to lab duties or specimen collection.

OSHA also requires all medical employers to train their staff about the dangers of bloodborne pathogens. Safety manuals must be available to guide you and other employees in the lab.

PERSONAL PROTECTIVE EQUIPMENT

OSHA also requires medical employers to provide workers with personal protective equipment (PPE). This reduces your chance of coming into contact with materials that might be hazardous. Here's what PPE you might need:

- latex or vinyl disposable gloves
- gown
- apron
- face shield
- goggles
- glasses with side shields
- mask
- lab coat
- shoe covers

PPE should fit the level of hazard to which you could be exposed. For example, when you're drawing blood or assisting with the collection of tissue samples, you should have disposable gloves. If you might encounter splashes or splatters, or an **aerosol** (particles suspended in gas or air), your eyes, face, and even your shoes should be covered.

> Let your employer know if you're allergic to latex. You can use latex-free PPE instead.

HazCom Standard

The HazCom Standard requires that all hazardous materials have a visible manufacturer's label. The label must include the following information:

- a warning, such as "DANGER"
- a statement of the specific hazard, such as "FLAMMABLE"
- precautions to follow to avoid exposure
- first aid measures to take if you're exposed

In addition, manufacturers must provide an MSDS for their products. The MSDS must include guidelines for safe storage, information about fire risk, and exposure precautions.

The standard requires employers to have written guidelines for handling each hazardous material in the workplace. This information should include the manufacturer's MSDS.

All this information should be available in a binder in the lab. You should review the MSDSs regularly to keep safety precautions and first aid procedures fresh in your mind.

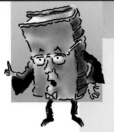

Legal Brief   FAILING TO FOLLOW OCCUPATIONAL SAFETY AND HEALTH ADMINISTRATION REGULATIONS

If your lab is not following OSHA rules, your health and the health of your coworkers could be in danger! In addition, the lab could be fined and all violations would have to be corrected. OSHA inspectors would revisit the lab to see if that had been done. If the lab failed to correct its problems, or continued to have other violations, it could even lose its license. In that case, it might have to close.

IT'S UP TO YOU

A medical laboratory can be a safe place to work—or it can be a not-so-safe place. Your daily behaviors and those of your coworkers will help determine which kind of place your lab will be. Here are some tips for making the lab a safe place to work, both for you and the people around you.

Personal Behaviors

Daily routine activities can affect lab safety. Here are some important guidelines for the lab.

- Never eat, drink, or smoke in the lab area.
- Never touch your face, mouth, or eyes with pens, pencils, or any other items used in the lab (including your gloves).
- Don't apply makeup or insert contact lenses in the lab.
- Wear glasses instead of contact lenses when working around chemicals that give off fumes.

Protect Yourself

Here are some precautions you should take to lessen your risk of exposure to lab hazards.

- Wear gloves whenever you may come in contact with blood, body fluids, secretions, excretions, broken skin, or mucous membranes.
- Wash your hands frequently. Always wash before and after gloving and before leaving the work site.
- If splatters, splashes, spills, or aerosols are a possibility, wear appropriate PPE. Use a splatter guard or splash shield whenever these risks exist.
- When opening a container, hold its mouth away from you and others to avoid aerosols, splashes, and spills.
- When removing a stopper, hold the opening away, use gauze around the cap, and twist gently. Avoid glove contact with the specimen.
- Avoid spills by pouring carefully. Pour at eye level if possible, but never near your face.

Protect Your Coworkers

Some of your work practices in the lab will make it a safer place to be. The following practices will protect both you and your coworkers.

- Store all chemicals according to the manufacturer's instructions.

Closer Look   SPILLS AND SPLATTERS

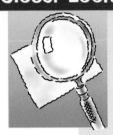

Spills, splatters, and exposure to aerosols are most likely to occur in these circumstances:

- taking the stopper off a blood collection tube
- transferring blood from a collection syringe to a specimen container
- conducting tests using the centrifuge
- preparing a smear

- Discard any container with an unreadable label.
- Label all specimen containers with biohazard labels.
- Place caps tightly on all containers immediately after use.
- Clean reusable glassware and other containers with recommended disinfectant or soap. Dry them thoroughly before using them again. (Wear gloves when washing and drying.)
- Disinfect all lab surfaces when you're finished using them and at the end of each day. Use a ten-percent bleach solution (nine parts water: one part bleach) or an appropriate disinfectant.
- Never allow clutter to accumulate.
- Dispose of needles and broken glass in sharps containers. Use biohazard containers to discard all other contaminated materials.

> Never store chemicals in unlabeled containers.

Be Informed and Prepared

Here are some other tips for preventing lab accidents and for being prepared in case one occurs.

- Read equipment manuals and know how to operate the equipment safely. Don't use damaged electrical equipment.
- Keep fire extinguishers close at hand. Many chemicals can catch fire and burn.
- Know the location and operation of all safety equipment, such as fire extinguishers, safety showers, and eyewash sta-

CLEANING UP SPILLS

Use proper procedures for removing chemical or biological spills. If the spill is chemical, follow the manufacturer's instructions on the MSDS. Commercial kits are available for such cleanups.

If the spill is biological, follow this procedure:

1. Put on gloves.

2. Cover the area with disposable material, such as paper towels, to soak up the spill. Discard the towels in a biohazard container.

3. Flood the area with disinfecting solution. Let the solution remain for 10 to 15 minutes.

4. Wipe up the solution and discard all waste in a biohazard container.

tions. (The illustration at right shows you how to use an eyewash station.)

• Immediately report any biohazard exposure or work-related injury to your supervisor.

Incident Reports

Whenever there's any kind of accident in a medical office, an incident report should be filled out. Of course, any exposure to a chemical or biological hazard should result in such a report. But here are some other times when an incident report is needed.

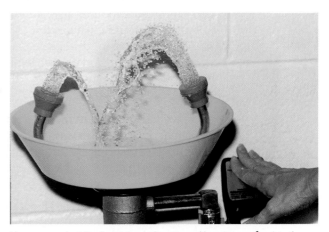

Use an eyewash station by turning on the water and lowering your face into the stream. Flush your eyes with the water until they are clear.

• An employee, patient, or visitor is stuck by a contaminated needle.

• A medication error takes place.

• Blood is drawn from the wrong patient.

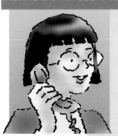

Ask the Professional ENFORCING SAFE PRACTICES

Q: *I've noticed that some of my coworkers sometimes don't wear gloves when handling slides and other specimens. I don't want to seem like a troublemaker, but this seems dangerous. Should I say something?*

A: You're right to be concerned. To some people, it may seem like a lot of trouble to wash their hands and use gloves every time they handle a specimen. But failing to do so not only risks that employee's health, it also endangers the health of everyone in the workplace—patients as well as workers.

Handwashing and wearing gloves helps protect employees from diseases caused by bacteria that might be present in the specimens they handle. More importantly, these precautions reduce the chances of spreading bacteria to other surfaces, where other employees or patients could come into contact with it.

One thing you can do is talk to the office or lab manager. Without mentioning any names, express your concern. The manager could call a meeting to remind all workers of the importance of following safe practices. If necessary, she also could monitor workers' behavior more closely.

The worker involved in the incident, or who was closest to the patient or visitor who was involved, should complete the report. Incident reports are important records, especially if the incident leads to some legal action against the office or lab.

Clinical Laboratory Improvement Amendments

Congress passed the **Clinical Laboratory Improvement Amendments** (CLIA) to improve the quality of medical testing in the United States. CLIA standards apply to all medical labs, from the largest reference labs to the smallest POLs. States also create their own rules for labs. These rules can be more strict than CLIA standards, but not less strict.

The CLIA program is carried out by two U.S. government agencies. They are the Centers for Medicare and Medicaid Services (CMS) and the Food and Drug Administration (FDA). CMS regulates the labs that conduct the tests. The FDA assigns each test to one of three categories, based on its level of difficulty.

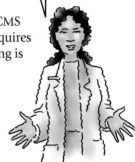

- *Waived tests.* These tests are the easiest to conduct and interpret. Many are simple enough for patients to do at home. Many POLs perform only waived tests.
- *Moderate-complexity tests.* POLs must be certified by CMS to perform these tests. The difficulty of these tests requires lab workers to have more training. Most of this testing is done in reference or hospital labs.
- *High-complexity tests.* Conducting and interpreting these tests requires high levels of training. They're rarely performed in POLs.

The table below shows examples of specific tests at each level.

> You can reference and download the most current list of waived tests from the CMS Web site at www.cms.hhs.gov/CLIA/.

PROVIDER-PERFORMED MICROSCOPY

Some moderate-complexity tests involve using procedures called provider-performed microscopy (PPM). POLs must have a special certificate from CMS to use PPM procedures.

Typical Lab Tests at Each Level of Testing

Waived	Moderate-Complexity	High-Complexity
• Dipstick urinalysis or reagent tablets • Fecal occult blood packets • Ovulation testing in packets with color comparison charts • Urine pregnancy test kits using color comparison charts • Manual erythrocyte sedimentation rate tests • Manual copper sulfate hemoglobin tests • Centrifuged micro-hematocrits • Blood glucose tests • Some rapid strep test kits • Flu kits	• Urine and throat cultures • Automated testing for cholesterol, high-density lipoproteins, and triglycerides • Gram staining • Microscopic urinalysis • Automated hematology with or without differential and no histogram • Manual white blood cell count differentials without identification of atypical cells • Automated coagulation tests that do not require intervention during analysis • Automated chemistry tests • Automated urinalysis tests	• Advanced cell studies (cytogenetics) • Cytology (such as Pap smears) • Histocompatibility • Histopathology • Manual cell counts

NOTE: CLIA is continually evaluating and changing methods for waived lab procedures. Always check the CMS Web site at www.cms.hhs.gov/CLIA/. If you find a test is waived by your method, print the document and save it.

They can be performed only by one of the following persons:

- physician
- dentist
- medical laboratory technologist
- nurse practitioner (under a physician's direct supervision)
- nurse midwife (under a physician's direct supervision)
- physician assistant (under a physician's direct supervision)

The PPM category includes the following tests:

- direct wet-mount preparations testing for bacteria, fungi, parasites, and cell properties
- potassium hydroxide preparations
- pinworm tests
- fern tests for amniotic fluid
- post-intercourse exams of vaginal or cervical mucous
- urine sedimentation exams
- nasal smear granulocytes
- fecal leukocytes
- semen analysis

If you're not sure about any test's category, you can check the CLIA Web site at www.fda.gov/cdrh/CLIA. An online search of CLIA's database will provide information about most of the tests performed in a lab.

Lab Standards

Each year, the CMS or the FDA may inspect labs that do moderate or high-complexity tests. These visits are unannounced. The inspectors show up without warning to check that the lab meets CLIA standards. They pay special attention to patient test management and quality control (QC).

Here are some things inspectors look for in judging patient test management.

- written standards of patient care and employee conduct
- clear policies and procedures for preparing patients and handling specimens

- a system to ensure that specimens are kept and identified properly for testing
- written procedures for performing tests, evaluating their safety and reliability, and handling questionable results
- a system to ensure that results are accurately recorded and reported

Of course, these safeguards all will be present if the lab has a good QC program.

QUALITY CONTROL (QC)

A good QC, program covers every part of the lab's performance. This includes making sure it measures up to required standards in the following areas:

- specimen collection and processing
- testing and reporting results
- reagents and equipment
- actual test performance
- personnel

Written procedures must exist to ensure that QC standards for monitoring test quality, accuracy, and reliability are in place.

Control Samples

Control samples are specimens provided by manufacturers. The contents of a control sample are known, so the outcome of the test performed on it is predictable.

Good QC procedures require testing control samples in these situations:

- *Each time a new reagent kit is opened.* This is to make sure the kit's materials are performing correctly. If the test results don't fall within the range given in the kit's package insert, the kit can't be used.
- *Each time the test is run on patient specimens.* This is a check on the accuracy of the patients' results. If the results on the control sample aren't in the range given in the test kit's package insert, the patient results can't be reported.

If the control sample test results fall outside the required range, here are the steps you should take.

1. Check the expiration dates of the reagent and control sample.
2. If the reagent has been prepared by mixing it with a liquid, check the mixture's accuracy and its expiration date.

3. Check that the testing equipment is clean and functioning accurately.

4. If all this has been done, remix the reagent or open a new reagent or control sample and test the control sample again.

Management of Reagents

Reagents are chemicals that produce a reaction. They each have a manufacturer's lot number and expiration date. You'll need to record these in your lab's QC log, as well as the dates the reagent was received and opened. If there's anything wrong with the reagent, the lot number and the dates can help the manufacturer identify the problem.

Instrument Calibration

Lab instruments should be handled gently and operated according to manufacturers' standards. Manufacturers also provide schedules for maintenance of their equipment. These schedules should be followed. All maintenance or repairs to equipment must be recorded in the QC log.

There are three components of instrument calibration.

- **Reportable range** is the range of tests an analyzer, instrument, or procedure is capable of producing results for. This is based on the machine's physical limitations, including light source, tubing, photo detectors, quality of chemicals, and others.

Closer Look   THE QUALITY CONTROL LOG

A lab must keep a QC log to show compliance with CLIA testing requirements. The log can be kept as a book or on the computer. It must include a record of each control sample and standard test. Here's what these entries must contain:

- the date and time of the test
- the results expected
- the results obtained
- the action taken for correction, if necessary

Your office must keep test records for two years. Records on maintenance of equipment and supplies also must be kept in the QC log.

- **Calibration** is setting the calculation points for the instrument by processing solutions of known values within the reportable range of the instrument. The solutions may or may not resemble clinical specimens. They may be measured quantities, a substance or standardized serum, or aqueous-based solutions.

- **Quality control specimens** are specimens that resemble clinical specimens. They have values that cover the calibrated range of the instrument. They may not exceed the upper or lower limits of the calibrated range. There are usually three levels—lower, middle, and upper. The QC specimens are selected to cover the expected range of patient results found in both healthy and sick patients. The controls have expected values and the instrument is expected to match these results plus or minus a small preset amount. The amount is known as *standard deviation.*

After you run the required controls for a procedure and they are all within acceptable ranges, you can report patient results with confidence. If they are not within acceptable ranges, the procedures and instruments must be evaluated. You must make the necessary changes and have acceptable QC results before you can rerun the tests and give the results to patients.

ALL ABOUT CALIBRATION

When calibrating an instrument, you must follow the exact directions of calibration. Solutions must be diluted in a certain way and sit for a specific amount of time. They also must be mixed for the correct time periods.

If a machine's calibration is correct and the control sample results fall within its reportable range, patient tests run on the machine will be correct.

Once they are ready to be processed through the instrument, there are even more rules that must be followed closely. Sometimes, these solutions may not be processed in the same way clinical specimens are processed through the instrument. This is different from quality control of instruments. When you perform quality control of an instrument, you process samples that resemble clinical specimens. The processing is identical to that used for clinical specimens.

When all of this is done correctly, this sets the value points an instrument will use to calculate values of unknown specimens.

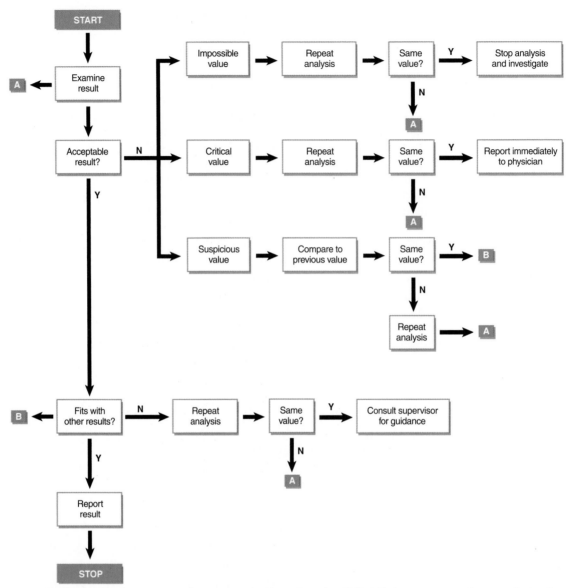

Following this flow chart helps prevent errors and inaccurate results. Y, yes; N, no. A and B (far left) show interconnection between evaluation of repeat testing and where decision-making strategy should resume. For example, if an impossible value is obtained and repeat analysis does not show the same value, the uppermost horizontal line of the chart says that the testing procedure should return to symbol A, where the steps are begun again with "Examine result."

Closer Look   QUALITY ASSURANCE

QC programs also must contain written policies and procedures to make sure lab employees meet the standards required by CLIA. Here are the ways the employer must do that.

- Determine each employee's educational background.
- Provide opportunities for continuing education and training.
- Conduct proficiency testing and use other methods to evaluate employees' competence.

Labs must keep a record of this information and make it available for inspection.

PROFICIENCY TESTING

Besides inspections, another way of finding out if a lab and its employees are competent is proficiency testing. Labs doing tests for patients who are covered by Medicare must take three proficiency tests each year. Here's how the program works.

- The lab receives specimens from an outside testing agency.
- The lab tests the specimens using the same methods it does for patient tests.
- The lab mails the results to the testing agency.
- The testing agency reviews the results and evaluates the lab's performance.

Medicare also requires labs to agree to at least one on-site inspection each year.

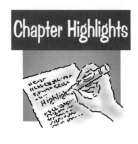

Chapter Highlights

- Labs perform tests that are key to diagnosing, preventing, and treating medical conditions and diseases. As a medical assistant, you'll have a critical role in this process.

- Large hospital labs and reference labs have specialized departments that perform complicated tests. The tests done in most physician office labs (POLs) are less complex.

- Microscopes, centrifuges, and chemical analyzers are basic equipment for lab tests. To ensure the accuracy of test results, they must be handled gently, operated correctly, and kept in good repair.

- The machinery, chemicals, and testing specimens in a lab can make it a hazardous place to work. These dangers can be reduced by following safe practices for the operation, storing, and handling of these items.

- OSHA rules set lab safety standards and procedures. CLIA standards regulate tests and testing methods. Failure to meet either set of requirements can have serious consequences.

- Good QC practices are basic to lab operations. These include careful control over reagents, test instruments, and test methods. They are also necessary for meeting CLIA requirements.

Chapter 2

PHLEBOTOMY

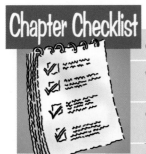

Chapter Checklist

- Identify the main methods of phlebotomy
- Identify equipment and supplies used in routine venipuncture and skin puncture
- List the major additives, their color codes, and the suggested order in which they are filled from a venipuncture
- Perform venipuncture and describe proper site selection and needle positioning
- Perform skin puncture
- Identify complications of venipuncture and skin puncture and how to prevent them
- Explain how to handle exposure to bloodborne pathogens

Physicians often analyze a patient's blood to help them determine the state of the patient's health. Blood tests can detect infections, as well as diabetes, heart disease, and many other conditions.

As a medical assistant, you may be responsible for collecting blood in your office. To make sure that diagnostic tests are accurate, you must collect these specimens in the correct way. You also must handle them according to accepted guidelines.

The Basics of Phlebotomy

The process of collecting blood is known as **phlebotomy.** The main methods for doing this are venipuncture and skin puncture. The name of each pretty much describes what is involved.

- In **venipuncture,** you use a hollow needle to puncture a large blood vessel called a **vein.** Small amounts of blood are withdrawn through the needle and sent to a lab for testing.
- In **skin puncture,** you pierce the skin with a sharp object. This causes **capillaries** (small blood vessels in the skin) to bleed, producing a specimen for testing.

BASIC BLOOD DRAWING EQUIPMENT

Both types of phlebotomy typically are performed at a blood drawing station. This is a place that is specially equipped for drawing blood. Here are the basic equipment and supplies you'll need there.

- *Table.* It should be high enough to reach easily and large enough to hold a variety of supplies.
- *Phlebotomy chair.* This special chair has adjustable armrests and safety locks to prevent falls in case of fainting.
- *Bed or reclining chair.* This should be available for patients with a history of fainting or for taking blood from infants and small children.
- *Gloves.* The Centers for Disease Control and Prevention (CDC) and the Occupational Health and Safety Administration (OSHA) require that gloves be worn when drawing blood.
- *Antiseptic.* **Antiseptics** block the growth of bacteria. The most common one used in blood collection is 70 percent isopropyl alcohol.
- *Gauze pads.* Two-by-two-inch gauze pads are used to hold pressure over the puncture site to stop the bleeding.
- *Bandages.* A small adhesive bandage is used to cover the puncture site once the bleeding has stopped.
- *Sharps containers.* These special containers are used to dispose of needles and other sharp objects.

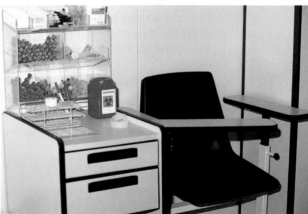

Venipuncture and skin puncture each have their own specialized

This well-stocked blood drawing station aids in the smooth performance of phlebotomy procedures.

equipment and methods. Let's look at equipment first and then turn to techniques.

> You'll need a new pair of gloves before drawing blood from each patient. Remove and discard them when you're finished.

VENIPUNCTURE EQUIPMENT

There are several methods for collecting blood by venipuncture. In general, they use the following equipment.

- *Tourniquet.* A tourniquet is a soft, flexible rubber strip that you wrap around the patient's arm to block the flow of blood in the veins. Doing this enlarges the veins, making them easier to find and puncture with a needle. You should use a new tourniquet for each patient.

- *Needles.* The needles used for drawing blood are hollow and coated with silicon so they will penetrate the skin smoothly. They are sterile, used only one time, and disposed of in a sharps container.

- *Evacuated tubes.* These containers hold the blood after it is drawn. They are made of glass or plastic and range in size from 2 to 15 milliliters (mL). A rubber stopper seals the end of the tube to protect the **vacuum** inside. (A vacuum is a space from which the air has been removed, or "evacuated.")

No matter which venipuncture method you use to draw blood, it will go the lab in these tubes.

Closer Look   NEEDLE GAUGES

Needles have different gauges. The **gauge** of a needle refers to the size of its opening, or lumen. The larger the gauge number, the smaller the opening of the needle. A 21- to 22-gauge needle is used for most blood collection. Choose a gauge that best fits the size and condition of the patient's vein. As you gain more experience with this process, you'll feel more confident choosing needle gauges. However, there are a few factors to consider when considering the condition of a patient's vein and which needle to choose.

- Veins in infants and the elderly may collapse under the normal vacuum of a normal size Vacutainer tube. The

(continued)

Closer Look   NEEDLE GAUGES (continued)

veins in infants and elderly patients may also be too small to accommodate the normal 20- or 21-gauge needle, so a smaller 23-gauge needle and smaller syringe should be used.

- The texture of an elderly patient's skin may be hard or scaly making it difficult to use a normal gauge needle, so a 23 should be used instead.

- Veins that are not straight are called tortuous veins. These veins may be easier to access with a 23-gauge needle.

- *Never* use a 24-gauge needle to collect blood, however. The opening is too small. This will cause **hemolysis,** or rupture of the blood cells

The Evacuated Tube System

The two collection methods most commonly used in venipuncture are the evacuated tube system and the syringe system.

The evacuated tube system has three parts:

- a multisample needle
- various collection tubes
- a plastic holder that attaches to the needle and holds the collection tubes

Using this system allows you to collect multiple tubes with a single venipuncture. It's a closed system. That means the

SHARPS WITH ENGINEERED SHARPS INJURY PROTECTION

OSHA has many regulations to promote safety in the medical office and to prevent needlestick injuries and blood-borne pathogen hazards. OSHA requires that all needles have a safety feature to reduce the risk of exposure. These *sharps with engineered sharps injury protection* are non-needles or needles with built-in safety features that prevent needle-sticks. These safety features should be simple and require little training to use effectively. They should also be activated using a one-handed behind-the-needle technique.

patient's blood flows from the vein through the needle and into the collection tube without exposure to air.

The illustration below shows an evacuated tube system's parts. The threaded hub on the multisample needle allows it to be screwed into the plastic holder. The tip of the longer part of the needle is cut on a slant or **bevel**. This lets it pierce the patient's skin and vein easily.

The needle's shorter end fits into a small hole in the holder and passes through the stopper of the collection tube. That end is covered by a rubber sleeve that is pushed back when it goes into the stopper. The large opening at the other end of the holder holds the blood collection tube. The rubber sleeve on the short end of the needle prevents leakage of blood during tube changes.

Choosing the Right Tube. The tube or tubes used in collecting the blood depends on a few things.

- The size of the tube and amount of vacuum in the tube can vary depending on the patient's age, amount of blood needed, and the condition of the patient's veins.

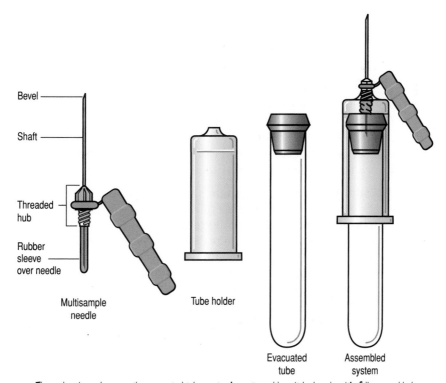

Bevel

Shaft

Threaded hub

Rubber sleeve over needle

Multisample needle

Tube holder

Evacuated tube

Assembled system

These drawings show you the evacuated tube system's parts and how it looks when it's fully assembled.

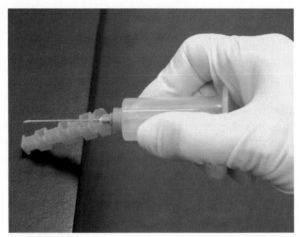

The Venipuncture Needle-Pro with needle resheathing device is an example of a safety tube holder.

The vacuum in each tube causes it to automatically fill with the amount of blood needed for that test. Larger tubes have more vacuum and draw blood through the needle faster. The speed that the blood passes through the tube can have an affect on the tests.

- The size of the tube also can depend on the amount of blood, serum, or plasma that is needed by the lab to perform the tests ordered.
- The color of the tube's stopper depends on the tests the physician orders. The tables on pages 41 and 59 explain the color-coding system.

In some cases, more than one tube of a given color may be required for the number of tests ordered.

Tube Additives. The color of a tube's stopper tells what additive the tube contains. An additive is a substance that is placed in the tube to affect the blood that is collected in it.

Different laboratory tests require different types of blood specimens. Some tests require serum samples. For these, the blood is drawn into a tube that contains nothing or a clot activator that speeds up clotting. Other tests require whole blood, or plasma. For these tests, blood is drawn into a tube that contains an additive to prevent clotting.

Here's a list of the most common additives and their functions.

- Anticoagulants prevent the blood from coagulating, or clotting.

(text continues on page 45)

Evacuated Tube System: Color Coding

BD Vacutainer™ Tubes with Hemogard™ Closure	BD Vacutainer™ Tubes with Conventional Stopper	Additive	Inversions at Blood Collection*	Laboratory Use	Your Lab's Draw Volume/ Remarks
		• Clot activator and gel for serum separation	5	BD Vacutainer™ SST™ Tube for serum determinations in chemistry. Tube inversions ensure mixing of clot activator with blood. Blood clotting time 30 minutes.	
		• Lithium heparin and gel for plasma separation	8	BD Vacutainer™ PST™ Tube for plasma determination in chemistry. Tube inversions prevent clotting.	
		• None (glass) • Clot activator (plastic tube with Hemogard closure)	0 5	For serum determinations in chemistry and serology. Glass serum tubes are recommended for blood banking. Plastic tubes contain clot activator and are not recommended for blood banking. Tube inversions ensure mixing of clot activator with blood and clotting within 60 minutes.	
		• Thrombin	8	For stat serum determinations in chemistry. Tube inversions ensure complete clotting which usually occurs in less than 5 minutes.	
		• Sodium heparin • Na_2EDTA • None (serum tube)	8 8 0	For trace-element, toxicology and nutritional-chemistry determinations. Special stopper formulation provides low levels of trace elements (see package insert).	

(continued)

Evacuated Tube System: Color Coding (*continued*)

BD Vacutainer™ Tubes with Hemogard™ Closure	BD Vacutainer™ Tubes with Conventional Stopper	Additive	Inversions at Blood Collection*	Laboratory Use	Your Lab's Draw Volume/ Remarks
		• Sodium heparin	8	For plasma determinations in chemistry.	
		• Lithium heparin	8	Tube inversions prevent clotting.	
		• Potassium oxalate/sodium fluoride	8	For glucose determinations. Oxalate and EDTA anticoagulants will give plasma samples.	
		• Sodium fluoride/ Na$_2$EDTA	8	Sodium fluoride is the antiglycolytic agent.	
		• Sodium fluoride (serum tube)	8	Tube inversions ensure proper mixing of additive and blood.	
		• Sodium heparin (glass)	8	For lead determinations. This tube is certified to contain less than .01 µg/ mL/(ppm) lead. Tube invasions prevent clotting.	
		• K$_2$EDTA (plastic)	8		
		• Sodium polyanethol sulfonate (SPS)	8	SPS for blood culture specimen collections in microbiology. Tube inversions prevent clotting.	
		• Acid citrate dextrose (ACD) additives:			
		Solution A— 22.0g/L trisodium citrate, 8.0g/L citric acid, 24.5g/L dextrose	8	ACD for use in blood bank studies, HLA phenotyping, DNA and paternity testing.	
		Solution B— 13.2g/L trisodium citrate, 4.8g/L citric acid, 14.7g/L dextrose	8		

BD Vacutainer™ Tubes with Hemogard™ Closure	BD Vacutainer™ Tubes with Conventional Stopper	Additive	Inversions at Blood Collection*	Laboratory Use	Your Lab's Draw Volume/ Remarks
		• Liquid K_3EDTA (glass) • Spray-dried K_2EDTA (plastic)	8 8	K_3EDTA for whole blood hematology determinations. K_2EDTA for whole blood hematology determinations and immuno-hematology testing (ABO grouping, Rh typing, antibody screening). Tube inversions prevent clotting.	
		• Spray-dried K_2EDTA	8	For whole blood hematology determinations and immunohematology testing (ABO grouping, RH typing, antibody screening). Designed with special cross-match label for re-quired patient information by the AABB. Tube inversions prevent clotting.	
		• .05M sodium citrate ($\approx$3.2%) • .129M sodium citrate (3.8%) • Citrate, theophylline, adenosine, dipyridamole (CTAD)	3–4 3–4 3–4	For coagulation determinations. NOTE: Certain tests may require chilled specimens. Follow your institution's recommended procedures for collection and transport. CTAD for selected platelet function assays and routine coagulation determination. Tube inversions prevent clotting.	

Partial-draw Tubes
(2 ml and 3 ml, 13 × 15 mm)

Small-volume Pediatric Tubes
(2 ml: 10.25 × 47 mm, 3 ml: 10.25 × 64 mm)

		• None	0	For serum determinations in chemistry and serology. Glass serum tubes are	

(*continued*)

BD Vacutainer™ Tubes with Hemogard™ Closure	BD Vacutainer™ Tubes with Conventional Stopper	Additive	Inversions at Blood Collection*	Laboratory Use	Your Lab's Draw Volume/ Remarks
				recommended for blood banking. Plastic tubes contain clot activator and are not recommended for blood banking. Tube inversions ensure mixing of clot activator with blood and clotting within 60 minutes.	
		• Sodium heparin	8	For plasma determinations in chemistry.	
		• Lithium heparin	8	Tube inversions prevent clotting.	
		• Liquid K_3EDTA (glass)	8	K_3EDTA for whole blood hematology determinations.	
		• Spray-dried K_2EDTA (plastic)	8	K_2EDTA for whole blood hematology determinations and immuno-hematology testing (ABO grouping, Rh typing, antibody screening). Tube inversions prevent clotting.	
		• .105M sodium citrate (=3.2%) • .129M sodium citrate (3.8%)	3–4	For coagulation determinations. Tube inversions prevent clotting. NOTE: Certain tests may require chilled specimens. Follow your institution's recommended procedures for collection and transport of specimen.	

BD Vacutainer Systems
Preanalytical Solutions
1 Becton Drive, Franklin Lakes, NJ 07417 USA. www.bd.com. *BD Technical Services:* 800.631.0174.
BD, BD Logo and all other trademarks are property of Becton, Dickinson and Company. ©2002 BD. Printed in USA 01/02 VS5229-4.
*Invert gently, do not shake.

- Clotting activators speed up coagulation so blood can be placed in a centrifuge sooner.
- Thixotropic gel separator forms a physical barrier between the cellular portion of a specimen and the serum or plasma portion after they have been separated by spinning the tube in a centrifuge.

You must use a tube with the correct colored stopper and the correct additive for each test the physician orders. The test results can be altered if you don't.

The Syringe System

Syringes are made of glass or disposable plastic. They vary in volume from 1 to 50 mL. When you choose a syringe, make sure it's big enough to hold enough blood for all the tests that have been ordered.

Pulling on the plunger of a syringe creates a vacuum in the barrel. The vacuum created by pulling on the plunger while a needle is in the patient's vein fills the syringe with blood. Pull the plunger slowly and rest between pulls so the vein has time to refill with blood.

After collecting blood in the syringe, you must transfer the blood into the evacuated tube for each test ordered. You should not apply force to the syringe plunger because the vacuum in the tube will draw the specimen from the syringe. Applying force may increase the chance of hemolysis.

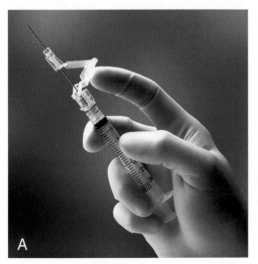
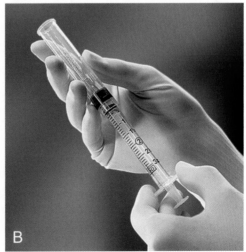

Here are two examples of syringes with safety features. (A) This is a syringe with a BD SAFETYGLIDE hypodermic needle attached. (B) This is the BD SAFETY-LOK Syringe SIMS Portex.

Secrets for Success

WORKING THE SYRINGE PLUNGER

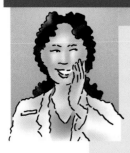

When you try to pull the plunger on a new syringe, the plunger may stick at first. This happens because the lubricant on the plunger forms a seal inside the barrel that must be broken for the plunger to move freely. You can make the plunger easier to move by using a technique called breathing the syringe. Before inserting the needle, pull back the plunger to about halfway up the barrel. Then push it back. Now the plunger will move more smoothly.

> It's very important to follow the proper order of draw when transferring blood from a syringe to an evacuated tube. You'll learn about the order of draw in this chapter.

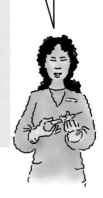

Winged Infusion Set

The winged infusion set, or the butterfly collection system, is used to collect blood from difficult or small veins. Examples might be veins in the hand or the veins of elderly patients or small children. This device consists of a stainless steel beveled needle with wing-shaped plastic extensions. These extensions are connected to a 6 to 12-inch length of tubing.

> The winged infusion set is also known as a butterfly set because the plastic extensions attached to the needle resemble butterfly wings.

The butterfly system can be used with either a syringe or an evacuated tube system. You'll need a multiple sample **Luer adapter** to connect the needle to the tube system. The photo on page 47 shows both types of setups. The photos on page 48 show how a winged infusion set is used.

SKIN PUNCTURE (MICROCOLLECTION) EQUIPMENT

There are times when venipuncture isn't the proper phlebotomy technique. Here are some examples.

- Only a few drops of blood are needed for the test.
- You don't want to make large blood draws from patients with small volumes of blood, such as infants.
- Some patients, such as those with extensive burns or scarring, may not have veins available for venipuncture.

In such cases, shallow punctures of the skin can be made, usually on the patient's fingers or heels, to obtain blood for testing. The equipment used to collect the specimen depends on the test being performed.

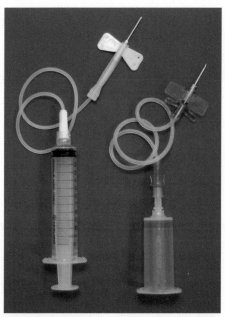

The winged infusion set on the left is attached to a syringe. The set on the right is attached to an evacuated tube holder using a multiple sample Luer adapter.

- *Lancets.* If drops of blood are needed for testing, you may use a sterile disposable lancet to pierce the skin. Lancets are designed to control depth of punctures. They also have safety features to reduce accidental sharps injuries. Lancets are available in a range of lengths and depths.
- *Microcollection containers.* Micro containers consist of plastic tubes and color-coded stoppers that show whether or not there is an additive in the tube. The color coding is the same as the coding on the blood collection tubes used in venipuncture. With a micro container, you can fill, measure, stopper, centrifuge, and store blood in one container.
- *Microhematocrit tubes.* These are small thin glass or plastic disposable tubes that fill by capillary action and hold 0.50 to 0.75 mL of blood. Blue hematocrit tubes are plain glass or plastic, and will clot if used to do a fingerstick hematocrit. Red hematocrit tubes are coated with an anticoagulant and won't clot when used for blood collected directly from a finger or heel.

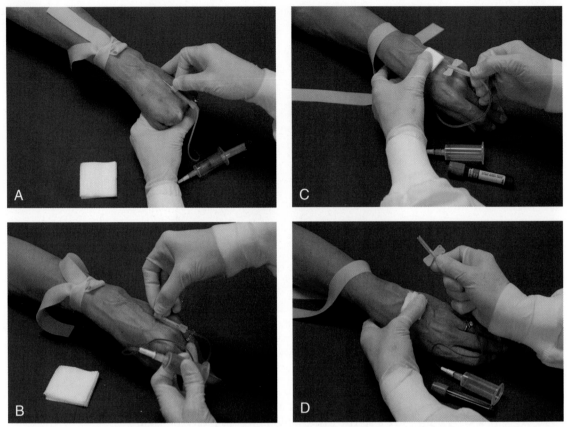

This is the procedure for using a butterfly in a hand vein. (A) Hand with tourniquet in place reveals prominent vein. (B) With the skin pulled taut over the knuckles, the needle is inserted into the vein until there is a "flash" of blood (about ⅛ of an inch) in the tubing. (C) Using the nondominant hand, one wing of the butterfly is held against the patient's hand to steady the needle while the blood collecting tube is pushed onto the blood-collecting needle. (D) Once the proper tubes have been drawn, gauze is placed over the vein, and the needle is removed.

Filter Paper Test Requisitions

Another microcollection device is filter paper that is part of a test requisition. This special filter paper is used to test newborns for genetic defects, such as hypothyroidism and phenylketonuria. The filter paper is printed with circles that must be filled with blood.

To use the paper test:

1. Clean the bottom lateral surface of the infant's heel with alcohol and wipe dry with a sterile gauze pad or allow to air dry.

2. Puncture the bottom lateral surface of the newborn's heel. Wipe away the first droplet with sterile gauze.

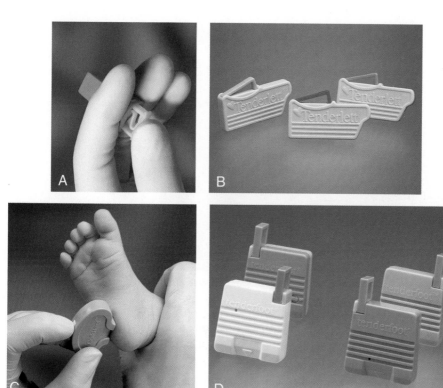

These photos show different types of finger and heel puncture lancets. (A) Vacutainer Genie Lancet. (B) Tenderlett toddler, junior, and adult lancet devices. (C) Becton Dickinson QuikHeel infant lancet. (D) Tenderfoot toddler, newborn, preemie, and micro-preemie heel incision devices.

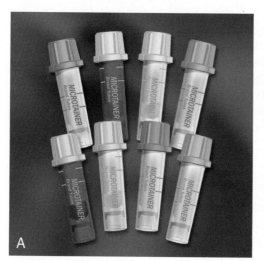

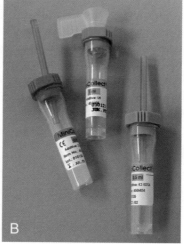

Here are some examples of microcollection containers: (A) Microtainers and (B) MiniCollect Capillary Blood Collection Tubes.

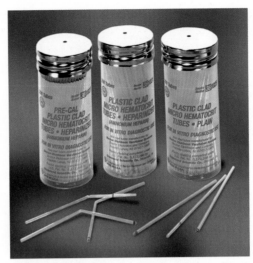

Microhematocrit tubes typically hold 0.50 to 0.75 mL of blood.

3. Allow a large blood droplet to form. Gently touch the circle on the filter paper against the droplet so it can be absorbed into the filter paper card.

4. Repeat, using a new droplet for each circle. Let the blood droplet soak through to the other side of the filter paper.

5. Allow the filter paper to air dry in a horizontal position. Do *not* stack with other collection requisitions.

Warming Devices

Warmers increase blood flow before the skin is punctured. This is especially important for heel sticks. Heel-warming devices provide a temperature not exceeding 42 degrees C or 105 degrees F.

Heel warmers are typically used only on infants. They may also be used on any individual with poor circulation. As an alternative, you can fill a latex glove with warm water. Then tie the opening in a knot.

Performing Phlebotomy

Some patients are anxious about having blood collected. Putting the patient at ease is part of the process. Here's how:

- Introduce yourself and explain the procedure in simple terms.
- Talk quietly and speak in a pleasant manner.
- Be cheerful and confident.

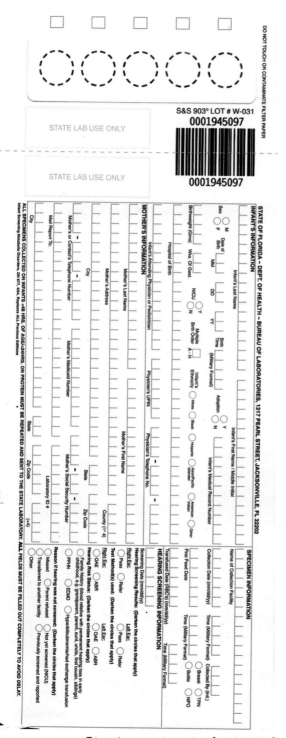

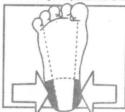

NEVER TOUCH FILTER PAPER CIRCLES
KEEP AWAY FROM ALL CONTAMINANTS

INSTRUCTIONS FOR COLLECTING BLOOD SAMPLE

1. Complete <u>ALL</u> information using a ballpoint.

2. Using appropriate blood handling precautions, clean infant's heel with alcohol swab. Dry area.

3. Puncture heel with appropriate sterile lancet (depth <2.4mm). Wipe away first drop with sterile gauze.

4. Allow large drop to form. Gently touch filter (circle) paper against large drop of blood, quickly allowing blood to soak through to fill circle. Do not press against heel. Apply to only one side of paper, saturating through to reverse side.

5. Using only one large drop per circle fill all circles. <u>EXAMINE BOTH SIDES TO ASSURE SATURATED, SINGLE DROP, NON-DAMAGED COLLECTION.</u>

6. Elevate infant's foot above body, pressing dry sterile pad or swab until bleeding stops.

7. Air dry in suspended horizontal position at least 3 hrs. at ambient temperature making sure that blood spots do not come into contact with anything until completely dry.

8. When completely dry, place into protective envelope.

9. Using pre-addressed mailing envelope, mail within 24 hrs. after collection.

See above diagram for puncture site. Place infant's limb in a position to increase venous pressure. Warming the skin-puncture site can increase blood flow through the site. A warm moist towel at a temperature no higher than 42°C may be used to cover the site for 3 minutes.

S&S 903® LOT # W-031

<u>ATTENTION: ALL PERSONNEL HANDLING INFANT SCREENING CARDS</u>

These new cards contain a <u>biohazard shield</u> which <u>must be flipped over the dried blood spot blotter before mailing</u> to the state laboratory.

Note: DO NOT USE THIS BIOHAZARD SHIELD AS A SURFACE FOR DRYING!

Please continue to dry the card flat and freely open to air on all sides.

This newborn screening specimen form shows the filter paper circles where blood should be absorbed.

Also make sure that you listen to the patient. Some patients know from experience where it is easiest to find an accessible vein.

> If you're using a latex glove filled with warm water instead of a commercial heel warmer, just be sure the water isn't too hot. You don't want to burn the patient.

BEFORE THE PROCEDURE

There are several steps you must take before you begin the actual collection of blood. First, you must identify the patient to be sure that you are collecting blood from the right person. Ask the patient to state:

- her name
- her date of birth
- any other information to verify identity

Next, check to see if the patient has followed any required dietary instructions or restrictions. The most common one is fasting. This requires the patient to avoid eating for a certain period, usually from midnight until the specimen is collected. If the patient indicates that she didn't follow the dietary restrictions, notify the physician. If you're told to proceed in obtaining the specimen, write "nonfasting" on both the test requisition and the specimen label.

> When instructing patients about fasting for a blood test, encourage them to drink water. Good hydration makes the veins more accessible for a draw.

PERFORMING A VENIPUNCTURE

Most often, you will use the forearm veins in the **antecubital space** (the inside of the elbow) for venipuncture. The three main veins in this area are:

- median cubital
- cephalic
- basilica

Your first choice should be the median cubital vein.

Applying a Tourniquet

As with any procedure, you should wash your hands and put on your gloves before applying a tourniquet. Here are the steps to follow.

1. When you're ready to apply the tourniquet, you should place it three to four inches above the site from which you plan to take blood.

2. Secure the tourniquet with a half-bow knot. Using this knot lets you rapidly remove the tourniquet with just

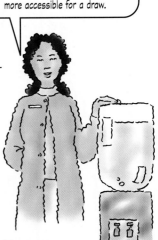

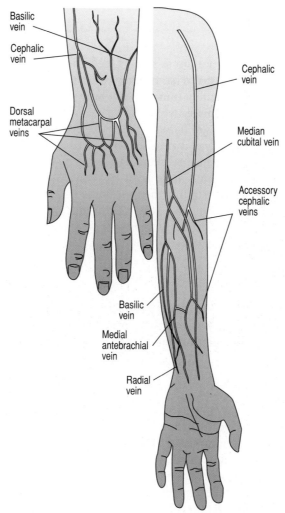

Left, Forearm, wrist, and hand veins subject to venipuncture. Right, Principal veins of the arm, including major antecubital veins subject to venipuncture.

one hand. Rapid removal is important. If it stays in place longer than one minute, the blood will change because of **hemoconcentration,** or the pooling of blood components.

3. Apply the tourniquet tightly enough to slow venous blood flow without affecting arterial blood flow. You will learn by experience how tight to put on a tourniquet by observing what tightness gets the best results on different patients.

Legal Brief PATIENT'S CONSENT TO COLLECT BLOOD

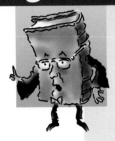

It's always important to respect the patient's rights. Even when the physician has ordered the collection of a blood sample, the patient must in some way give his consent to it. Rolling up his sleeve would be one way of showing consent. This is called *implied consent* because the action suggests or *implies* that he's willing to cooperate. It's better, however, to get a direct verbal consent, also known as *expressed consent*. Simply ask the patient, "Are you ready to begin?" before starting the procedure. If you go ahead without obtaining the patient's consent, and he objects, you could be charged with assault and battery.

4. Ask the patient to make a fist. Do NOT allow the patient to open and close the fist because this will also cause hemoconcentration and lead to inaccurate test results.

The illustration on page 55 shows how the tourniquet should be applied.

Site Selection

Use the tip of your index finger to **palpate,** or feel, veins to select a vein for puncture. Palpating helps locate veins and determine their size, depth, and direction. To palpate a vein, extend your index finger and touch the patient's skin with the soft pad at the end of the finger. Then rapidly and repeatedly "bounce" this finger on the patients skin about ⅛ of an inch above the surface in the area you expect to find a vein. Moving in a side-to-side progression, you should go across a patient's arm. When you have crossed the arm, move down the arm about a ¼ inch and go back in the opposite direction. When you feel what you think is a vein, you can attempt to trace the vein by palpitation. The depth is determined by experience and palpitation.

A good vein should be

- straight for one or more inches
- engorged in blood sufficiently to make it prominent and firm
- surrounded by sufficient tissue to keep it in place

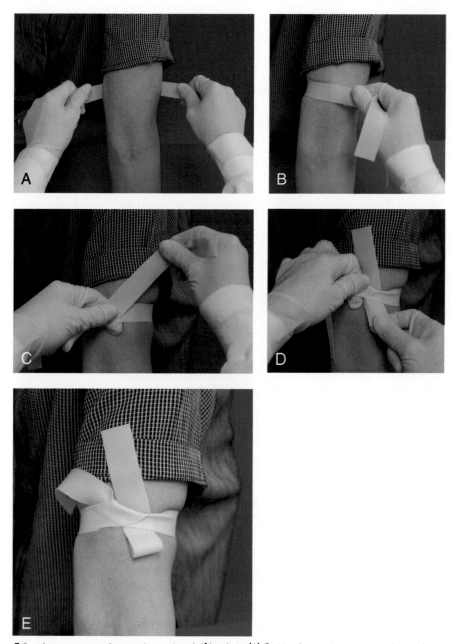

Follow these steps to apply a tourniquet using a half-bow knot. (A) Position the tourniquet as you see here and apply tension. (B) Grasp both tourniquet sides between thumb and forefinger of right hand. (C) Cross the left side of tourniquet over the right side with both sides held between thumb and index finger of the left hand. (D) Tuck the left end of tourniquet under right side, forming a loop. (E) This is how a properly tied tourniquet should look.

- located in an area with no hematoma
- under skin that is soft and clear of abnormalities

If you can't find a good vein on one arm, release the tourniquet and repeat the procedure on the other arm. If you can't locate a suitable antecubital vein on either arm, check hand veins and finally wrist veins. You can try massaging the arm from wrist to elbow to increase blood flow and make veins more palpable. You also can use a warm towel to do the same thing.

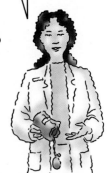

A Velcro strap, rubber tubing, or even a blood pressure cuff can be used as a tourniquet for drawing blood.

Needle Positioning

If you can't obtain blood once you've punctured a vein, you may have to change the needle's position. The illustration on page 57 shows proper and improper placements of the needle.

Running Smoothly   BLOOD DRAWS AND FAINTING

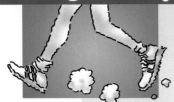

What do I do if a patient feels faint during a blood draw?

You're busy drawing blood when the patient says he feels faint. You must respond immediately. Follow these steps to keep the patient safe.

1. Remove the tourniquet and take out the needle as quickly as possible.

2. Talk to the patient to distract him from the procedure and to help keep him alert.

3. Have the patient lower his head and breathe deeply. You should physically support the patient to protect him if he does collapse.

4. Loosen a tight collar or tie if possible.

5. Put a cold compress or washcloth on his forehead and on the back of his neck.

6. Call for the physician if the patient doesn't respond.

Always believe patients who tell you in advance that they faint during venipuncture. For safety, ask these patients to lie down during the procedure. This reduces the chance of **syncope** (fainting). It also ensures that the patient won't fall if he or she does faint. Never draw blood from a patient who is likely to faint unless the physician is in the office.

Here are some of the common problems with needle position:

- The needle may be against the wall of the vein. Correct by rotating the needle half a turn.

- The needle may not have penetrated the vein. Correct by slowly advancing the needle farther into the vein.

- The needle may have penetrated too far into the vein. Correct by pulling it back a little.

- The tube may not have sufficient vacuum. Correct by trying another tube before withdrawing the needle.

Never attempt a venipuncture more than twice. If you can't obtain a specimen in two tries, have another person attempt the draw, or perform a skin puncture if possible.

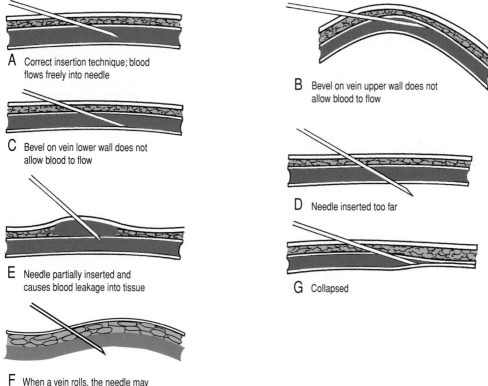

A Correct insertion technique; blood flows freely into needle

B Bevel on vein upper wall does not allow blood to flow

C Bevel on vein lower wall does not allow blood to flow

D Needle inserted too far

E Needle partially inserted and causes blood leakage into tissue

G Collapsed

F When a vein rolls, the needle may slip to the side of the vein without penetrating it

Proper and improper needle positioning. (A) Needle correctly positioned in a vein; blood flows freely into the needle. (B) Needle bevel on the upper wall of the vein prevents blood flow. (C) Needle bevel on the lower wall of the vein prevents blood flow. (D) Needle inserted too deep runs through the vein. (E) Partially inserted needle causes blood to leak into tissue. (F) Needle slipped beside the vein, not into it; occurs when a vein rolls to the side. (G) Collapsed vein prevents blood flow.

Order of Draw

The Clinical and Laboratory Standards Institute (CLSI) recommends the order in which evacuated tubes should be collected or filled from a syringe. The table on page 59 summarizes this information for you. It's important to follow order-of-draw guidelines to avoid any contamination of the specimens.

After you collect the specimens, label each tube with:

- the patient's first and last name
- an assigned identification number if available
- the date and time
- your initials to verify that you drew the sample

PERFORMING A SKIN PUNCTURE

Many blood tests are more accurate when conducted on the larger specimens obtained through venipuncture, although technology now allows some tests to be performed on very small samples. This lets you obtain capillary samples by doing skin punctures.

Skin puncture is the preferred way of getting blood from children and infants. Performing venipuncture on such patients can damage their veins and surrounding tissues. Also, restraining the infant or child might cause injury.

When you're collecting blood by skin puncture from an adult, choose either the middle or ring finger because they are less calloused than the forefinger.

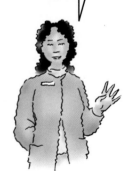

You might perform a skin puncture on an adult patient:

- when no veins are accessible
- to save veins for procedures such as chemotherapy
- for point-of-care testing, or any testing done outside of a designated laboratory or blood drawing area, for example, in an exam room. The most common point-of-care testing is glucose testing.

The Hands On feature on page 70 provides the step-by-step procedure for performing a skin puncture.

When Things Go Wrong

Phlebotomy is a skill that requires specialized knowledge, practice, and attention to detail. Errors can be made during the preparation for the procedure, during the procedure, or after the procedure is complete.

The table on page 60 lists some of the mistakes commonly made in doing venipunctures and skin punctures. Pay attention to the ways in which errors are made so you can guard against making them yourself.

Order of Draw, Stopper Color, and Rationale for Collection Order

Order of Draw	Tube Stopper Color	Rationale for Collection Order
Blood cultures (sterile collections)	Yellow sodium polyan-etholesulfonate (SPS) (or sterile media containers)	• Minimizes chance of microbial contamination
Plain (nonadditive) tubes	Red	• Prevents contamination by additives in other tubes
Coagulation tubes	Light blue	• Second or third position in order of draw prevents tissue thrombo-plastin contamination • Must be the first additive tube in the order because all other additive tubes affect coagulation tests
Serum separator gel tubes (STS)	Red and gray rubber; gold plastic	• Prevents contamination by additive in other tubes • Comes after coagulation tests because silica particles activate clotting and affect coagulation tests; carryover of silica into subsequent tubes can be over-ridden by the anticoagulant in them
Plasma separator gel tubes (PSTs)	Green and gray rubber; light green plastic	• Contains heparin, which affects coagulation tests and interferes in collection of serum specimens • Causes the least interference in tests other than coagulation tests
Heparin tubes	Green	• Same as PST
Ethylenediamine-tetraacetic acid (EDTA) tubes	Lavender	• Causes more carryover problems than any other additive • Elevates sodium and potassium levels • Chelates and decreases calcium and iron levels • Elevates prothrombin time and partial thromboplastin time results
Oxalate/fluoride tubes	Gray	• Sodium fluoride and potassium oxalate elevate sodium and potas-sium levels, respectively • Comes after hematology tubes because oxalate damages cell membranes and causes abnormal red blood cell morphology

COMPLICATIONS OF VENIPUNCTURE

You must be careful when drawing blood because of the risks involved in venipuncture. These include nerve damage, artery puncture, hematoma formation, and skin infection.

Common Sources of Error in Phlebotomy

Sources of Error in Venipuncture

Errors in Preparation	Errors in Procedure	Errors After Completion
• Improper patient identification • Failure to check patient adherence to dietary restrictions • Failure to calm patient prior to blood collection • Use of improper equipment and supplies • Inappropriate method of blood collection	• Failure to dry site completely after cleansing with alcohol • Inserting needle bevel side down • Use of needle that is too small, causing hemolysis of specimen • Venipuncture in an unacceptable area • Prolonged tourniquet application • Wrong order of tube draw • Failure to mix blood collected in additive-containing tubes immediately • Pulling back on syringe plunger too forcefully • Failure to release tourniquet prior to needle withdrawal	• Failure to apply pressure immediately to venipuncture site • Vigorous shaking of anticoagulated blood specimens • Forcing blood through a syringe needle into tube • Mislabeling of tubes • Failure to label appropriate specimens with infectious disease precaution • Failure to put date, time, and initials on requisition • Slow transport of specimens to laboratory

Sources of Error in Skin Puncture

Errors in Preparation	Errors in Procedure	Errors After Completion
• Misidentification of patient	• Puncturing wrong area of infant heel • Puncturing bone in infant heel • Puncturing fingers of infants • Puncturing wrong area of adult finger • Contaminating specimen with alcohol or Betadine • Failure to discard first blood drop • Collecting air bubbles in pH or blood gas specimen • Excessive massaging of puncture site • Bruising site as a result of excessive squeezing	• Hemolyzing specimen • Failure to seal specimens adequately • Failure to chill specimens requiring refrigeration • Erroneous specimen labeling • Failure to document skin puncture collection on the requisition or in the computer • Delaying specimen transport

Permanent nerve damage can result from:

- poor site selection
- movement of the patient during needle insertion
- inserting the needle too deeply or quickly
- excessive blind probing

Another possibly serious complication of venipuncture is the puncture of an artery. You'll know this has happened by the blood's bright red color and the pulsing of the specimen into the tube. If you accidentally puncture an artery, hold pressure over the site for a full five minutes after the needle is removed and apply a pressure bandage. A pressure bandage is made by folding a two-by-two-inch gauze twice to quarter it. It is placed over the venipuncture site and then covered with a bandage.

The most common complication of venipuncture is **hematoma** formation. This happens when blood leaks into the tissues during or after the draw. Hematomas may be painful and may cause unsightly bruising. In rare incidences, they also can cause compression injuries to nerves.

If a hematoma begins to form during the draw, follow these steps.

1. Release the tourniquet immediately.
2. Withdraw the needle.
3. Hold pressure on the site for at least two minutes.
4. Apply cold compresses to reduce the pain and swelling.

You can prevent another possible complication, the infection of the site, by following these antiseptic techniques.

- not touching the site after cleaning
- removing the needle cap at the last possible minute prior to venipuncture
- not opening bandages ahead of time

PREVENTING HEMATOMAS

The following situations can trigger hematoma formation. Being aware of them will help you prevent hematomas from forming in your patients.

- The vein is fragile or too small for the needle.
- The needle is only partly inserted into the vein.
- Excessive or blind probing is used to find the vein.
- The needle is removed while the tourniquet is still on.
- Pressure isn't adequately applied after venipuncture.

COMPLICATIONS OF SKIN PUNCTURE

It can be difficult to obtain a skin puncture specimen without clots. This is because the body's clotting system works to stop bleeding as soon as the skin is punctured. Therefore, blood should be drawn in a specific order.

1. First, collect an anticoagulated specimen before blood begins to clot.
2. Next, collect any other additive specimens.
3. Last, collect clotted specimens.

BLOOD EXPOSURE SAFETY

You must be extremely careful when collecting specimens. Blood is a hazardous material. Handle blood using standard precautions. Needlestick injuries can expose you to blood-borne pathogens, such as hepatitis B, hepatitis C, and human immunodeficiency virus (HIV). Your risk of infection depends on:

- the pathogen you were exposed to
- the severity of the needlestick injury

Ask the Professional   **FOLLOWING BLOOD DRAW PROCEDURES**

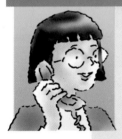

Q: *I've noticed that one of my coworkers is not following the proper procedures for blood draw. I feel like I should say something, but we are friends outside of work. I want to keep our friendship. What should I do?*

A: Yes, you should talk with your coworker. It may be uncomfortable for you, but remember that you're a medical professional and you must act like one. You have a legal and ethical responsibility to make sure patients get the best possible care. Talk to your friend at a time when both of you are relaxed. Tell her that you've noticed she's not following the blood draw procedure you learned and that you'd like to help. Be willing to listen to her side of the situation and give her the benefit of the doubt. She may be unsure of the proper procedures to follow.

If you find that your coworker has not corrected the problem after you have talked, then you should talk to your supervisor.

- whether you were vaccinated before you were exposed
- **prophylaxis** (protective treatment for the prevention of disease once you've been exposed)

Make sure you know what to do if you have a needlestick accident or other exposure.

Cleaning up Spills

Accidents do happen. As a medical assistant, you must know how to clean up spills of blood or other body fluids. Here's what to do:

1. Secure the spill area.
2. Locate a spill cleanup kit.
3. Wear gloves during cleanup.
4. Pour or place absorbent material over the spill.
5. Use a scoop or dustpan to pick up material.
6. Wipe up fluids with an absorbent towel.
7. Apply a disinfectant to the area.
8. Double-bag all cleanup materials in red biohazard bags for disposal.

When cleaning up spills of any body fluid, make sure you use disposable gloves that will not tear during cleaning. If your gloves develop holes, tears, or slits, remove them and wash your

HANDLING A SHARPS INJURY OR EXPOSURE TO BODY FLUIDS

If you have a sharps injury or are exposed to a patient's blood or body fluids, you must take immediate action. Follow these steps to protect yourself.

- Wash the needlestick area and cuts with soap and water.
- Flush splashes to the nose, mouth, or skin with water.
- Irrigate eyes with clean water, saline, or sterile irrigant.
- Report the incident to your supervisor.
- Immediately seek medical treatment.

To protect yourself and others, immediately dispose of used needles, lancets, and other sharp objects into a sharps container.

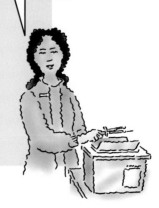

hands immediately. Then put on fresh gloves to finish cleaning up the spill. Never wash or reuse disposable gloves.

Spills should be properly cleaned using a hospital-approved chemical disinfectant or a solution of household bleach diluted 1:10 with water. Here are some steps you should take first if there is glass from broken evacuated tubes with the blood.

1. Wear double gloves or utility gloves.
2. Pick up the glass with forceps, or scoop it up with a broom and dustpan or cardboard. *Never* use your hands to pick up the glass.
3. Place the broken glass in a sharps container.
4. Then follow the other steps for cleaning up a blood or body fluid spill.

The Biohazard Spill Kit

Your medical office should always have a biohazard spill kit on hand. This kit should contain the following supplies:

- biohazard spill cleanup instructions
- nitrile disposable gloves
- laboratory coat or impervious apron
- absorbent material, such as absorbent paper towels and granular absorbent material
- all-purpose disinfectant such as normal household bleach (diluted 1:10) or a hospital disinfectant
- bucket for diluting disinfectant (can be used to store kit supplies when not in use), if required
- dustpan, broom, hand broom (for picking up broken glass and contaminated sharps)
- sharps waste containers
- biohazard waste bags

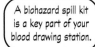

A biohazard spill kit is a key part of your blood drawing station.

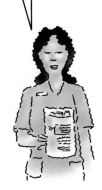

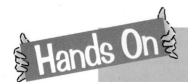

OBTAINING A BLOOD SPECIMEN BY VENIPUNCTURE

2-1

To perform a venipuncture, you'll need the following equipment: needle, syringe, and test tubes or evacuated tubes; tourniquet; sterile gauze pads; bandages; needle and adaptor; sharps container; 70-percent alcohol pad or other antiseptic; permanent marker or pen; and biohazard barriers such as gloves, impervious gown, and face shield.

Follow these steps to perform venipuncture.

1. Check the requisition slip to see what tests have been ordered. Also note the specimen requirements.

2. Assemble your equipment. Don't use any equipment that has expired.

3. Wash your hands.

4. Greet and identify the patient. Explain the procedure and answer any questions. If the patient was required to fast, ask how long it's been since she ate. (It should have been at least eight hours.)

5. Put on nonsterile latex gloves. Follow standard precautions.

6. Get your needle ready by following procedures for using a syringe or an evacuated tube.

7. Ask the patient to sit with a well-supported arm. Veins in the antecubital fossa are easiest to locate when the arm is straight to a 15-degree bend at the elbow.

8. Apply the tourniquet around the patient's arm three to four inches above the elbow. Check that it is snug but not too tight. Secure by using a half-bow knot. Make sure the tails of the tourniquet go toward the shoulder. Ask the patient to make a fist. Tell her to hold the fist and not to pump it.

9. Using your gloved index finger, palpate to find a vein. Then trace the vein with your finger.

10. Release the tourniquet.

11. Cleanse the venipuncture site with an alcohol pad. Allow it to dry or dry with sterile gauze. Don't touch the site after cleansing.

12. If you're drawing blood for a blood culture, be sure the specimen is sterile. You can do this by applying alcohol to the area. Then apply a two-percent iodine solution. Cover

(continued)

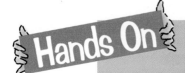

Hands On

OBTAINING A BLOOD SPECIMEN BY VENIPUNCTURE (*continued*)

2-1

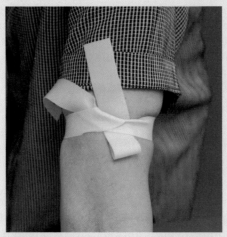

Use a half-bow to tie the tourniquet. Be sure it extends upward to avoid contaminating the venipuncture site.

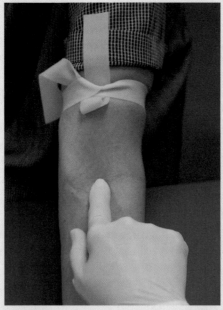

You should trace the vein with your gloved index finger to judge its depth.

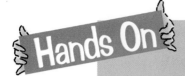

Hands On

OBTAINING A BLOOD SPECIMEN BY VENIPUNCTURE (*continued*)

2-1

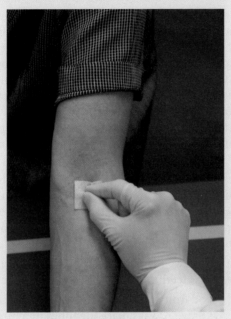

Cleanse the site with an alcohol pad.

the clean area with a sterile four-by-four-inch gauze pad for two minutes.

13. Now reapply the tourniquet. Ask the patient to make a fist. The maximum time the tourniquet should be in place is one minute.

14. You're ready to penetrate the vein. It's easier to do if you hold the syringe or assembly in your dominant hand. Grasp the patient's arm with the other hand and use your thumb to draw the skin taut over the site.

15. With the bevel up, line up the needle with the vein about one-fourth to one-half inch below the site where the vein is to be entered. Insert the needle into the vein at a 15- to 30-degree angle. Remove your nondominant hand and slowly pull back the plunger of the syringe. Or place fingers on the flange of the adapter and with the thumb push the tube

(*continued*)

Hands On

onto the needle inside the adapter. When blood begins to flow into the tube or syringe, you can release the tourniquet and allow the patient to release the fist. Allow the syringe or tube to fill to capacity. When blood flow stops, remove the tube from the adapter by gripping the tube with your non-dominant hand and placing your thumb against the flange during removal. Twist and gently pull out the tube. Hold the needle steady in the vein, without pulling up or pressing down, and insert any other necessary tubes into the adapter and fill each to capacity.

16. Remove the tube from the adapter *before* removing the needle from the arm. This is important because you don't want any blood to drip from the tip of the needle onto the patient. Place a sterile gauze pad over the puncture site as you are withdrawing the needle.

17. Apply pressure or have the patient apply direct pressure for five minutes. Don't let the patient bend the arm at the elbow.

18. Transfer the blood from the syringe into the tubes using the proper order of draw. Always place the tubes in a tube rack to do the transfer. If the tubes contain an anticoagulant, you should mix immediately by gently inverting the tube eight to ten times. Do not shake the tube. Label the tubes with the proper information.

19. Check the puncture site to be sure it isn't bleeding. Apply a dressing, a clean two-by-two-inch gauze pad that you've folded in quarters. Secure it with an adhesive bandage or three-inch strip of tape.

20. Thank your patient when you've finished. Tell your patient to leave the bandage in place for at least 30 minutes.

21. To finish your task, take care of or dispose of equipment and supplies. Clean your work area. Then you can remove your gloves and wash your hands.

22. Test, transfer or store the blood according to your office's policy.

23. Record the procedure.

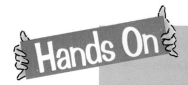

OBTAINING A BLOOD SPECIMEN BY VENIPUNCTURE (*continued*)

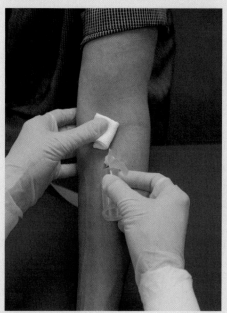

Do not apply any pressure to the puncture site until the needle is completely removed.

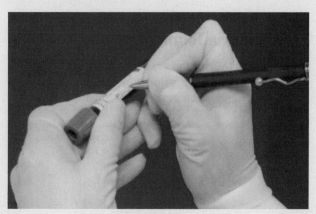

Label the tube with the necessary information.

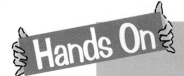

OBTAINING A BLOOD SPECIMEN BY SKIN PUNCTURE

2-2

To perform a skin puncture, you'll need the following equipment: sterile disposable lancet or automated skin puncture device; 70-percent alcohol or other antiseptic; sterile gauze pads; microcollection tubes or containers; heel-warming device (if necessary); and biohazard barriers such as gloves, impervious gown, and face shield.

Follow these steps to perform a skin puncture.

1. Check the requisition slip to see what tests have been ordered. Also note the specimen requirements.

2. Assemble your equipment.

3. Wash your hands.

4. Greet and identify the patient. Explain the procedure and answer any questions.

5. Put on gloves. Follow standard precautions.

6. Select the puncture site. It will be one of the following:

    (A) just off center of the tip of the middle or ring finger of the nondominant hand

    (B) the lateral curved surface of the heel

    (C) the heel of an infant

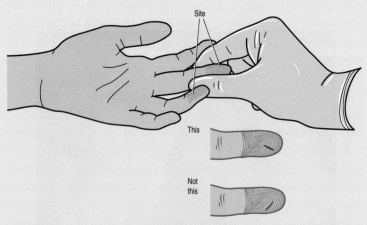

Make the finger puncture in the fleshy portion of the fingertip, just to the side of the center, and perpendicular to the grooves of the fingerprint.

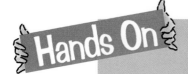

OBTAINING A BLOOD SPECIMEN BY SKIN PUNCTURE (*continued*)

2-2

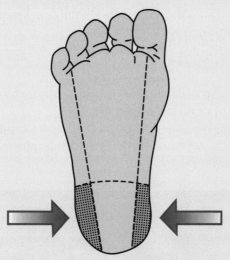

These areas of a newborn's heel are acceptable for puncture.

7. Make sure the site you've chosen is warm. Gently massage the finger from the base to the tip to increase the blood flow.

8. You'll use both hands for this procedure. Grasp the finger or heel firmly with your nondominant hand. Now cleanse the area with alcohol and wipe dry.

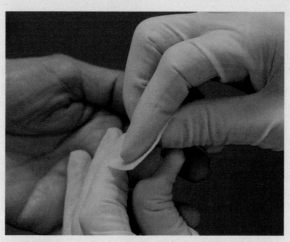

Cleanse the site with alcohol before performing the skin puncture.

(*continued*)

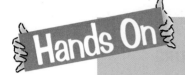

**OBTAINING A BLOOD
SPECIMEN BY SKIN PUNCTURE**
(*continued*)

2-2

9. While you hold the finger or heel firmly, make a swift, firm puncture using your dominant hand.
   - After puncture, dispose of the used puncture device in a sharps container.
   - Wipe away the first drop of blood. It may be contaminated with tissue fluid or residue from your alcohol wipe.
   - Apply pressure toward the site.

10. Collect the specimen. You can encourage blood flow by holding the puncture site downward and applying gentle pressure near the site.

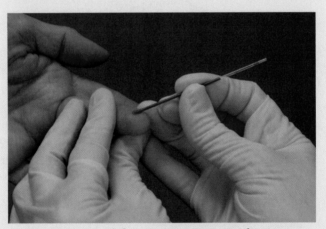

Touch only the tip of the collection tube to the drop of blood.

11. Once you've collected the blood you need, apply clean gauze to the site with pressure or have the patient apply pressure. Don't release your patient until the bleeding has stopped. Label the containers with the proper information.

12. Thank your patient when you've finished. Tell your patient to leave the bandage in place for at least 30 minutes.

13. To finish your task, take care of or dispose of equipment and supplies. Clean your work area. Then you can remove your gloves and wash your hands.

14. Test, transfer, or store the specimen according to your office's policy, and record the procedure.

Chapter Highlights

- A blood drawing station has the supplies and equipment needed for phlebotomy procedures.
- The venipuncture systems are the evacuated tube system and the syringe system.
- Venipuncture uses color-coded stoppers to identify the additive content of each type of tube.
- Blood specimens collected by venipuncture must be placed in evacuated tubes in proper order of draw.
- Lancets are used to pierce the skin to collect drops of blood in skin puncture.
- It's essential to identify the patient before performing a venipuncture or skin puncture.
- Hematoma is the most common complication of venipuncture.

Chapter 3

HEMATOLOGY

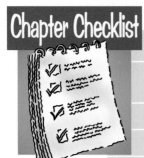

Chapter Checklist

- Explain the functions of the three types of blood cells
- Identify the leukocytes normally seen in the blood and explain their functions
- Describe the role of the hematology lab
- List the different tests in a complete blood count
- Specify the normal ranges for each test in a complete blood count
- Use a Unopette system to prepare a whole blood dilution
- Make a peripheral blood smear
- Stain a peripheral blood smear
- Perform a white blood cell differential
- Describe the structure of red blood cells and explain the tests that are performed on the cells
- Perform a manual microhematocrit determination
- Determine a Westergren erythrocyte sedimentation rate
- Explain the functions of platelets
- Explain the process of how blood clots form in the body and describe the tests that measure the ability to form clots

Hematology is the study of blood, blood-forming tissues, and blood diseases. In this chapter, you'll learn the vital role that blood plays in our overall health and how it is often used to perform important tests and diagnose illnesses. In addition to learning about blood tests used for diagnostic purposes, you'll also learn about coagulation tests used to monitor patients undergoing certain treatments. It may not always fall within your scope of practice as a medical assistant to perform certain tests or to analyze specimens. However, you'll need to be familiar with these tests and the techniques involved to prepare specimens that are usable.

Blood Basics

Blood is made of two parts—fluid (also known as plasma) and three basic types of cells:

- **leukocytes**, commonly called white blood cells or WBCs
- **erythrocytes**, commonly called red blood cells or RBCs
- **thrombocytes**, also known as platelets

The illustration on page 76 shows what each type of cell looks like under a microscope.

LEUKOCYTES

Leukocytes are the body's main line of defense against bacteria and viruses. There are three main kinds of leukocytes:

- lymphocytes
- monocytes
- granulocytes

Granulocytes can be further divided into these types of cells:

- neutrophils
- eosinophils
- basophils

ERYTHROCYTES

Red blood cells, or erythrocytes, carry gases between the lungs and the body's tissues. These gases are mainly oxygen and carbon dioxide. **Hemoglobin** molecules in each red blood cell carry these gases.

THROMBOCYTES

Platelets aren't actually cells. Instead, they're cell fragments. Their main function is to help stop bleeding. You'll read more about platelets and all the other types of cells later in the chapter. You'll also learn how each type is tested to judge a patient's health and identify disease.

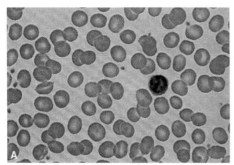

A blood smear enables blood cells to be examined under a microscope.

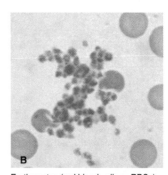

Erythrocytes (red blood cells or RBCs) are the large, round cells. The platelets have been stained purple.

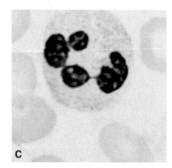

This segmented neutrophil is the most abundant of the leukocytes (white blood cells or WBCs).

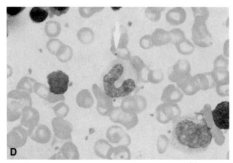

A neutrophil band is a younger, less mature version of the neutrophil.

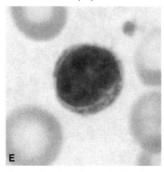

The lymphocyte is the smallest of the leukocytes (WBCs).

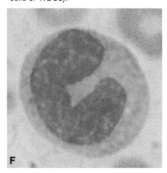

The monocyte is the largest of the normal WBCs with a less dense nucleus and slate gray (or blue gray) cytoplasm.

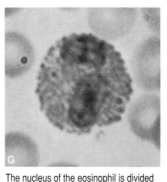

The nucleus of the eosinophil is divided into two parts.

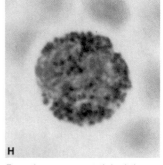

Fewer than one percent of circulating WBCs are basophils.

(A) A blood smear enables blood cells to be examined under a microscope. (B) Erythrocytes (red blood cells or RBCs) are the large, round cells. The platelets have been stained purple. (C) This segmented neutrophil is the most abundant of the leukocytes (white blood cells or WBCs). (D) A neutrophil band is a younger, less mature version of the neutrophil. (E) The lymphocyte is the smallest of the leukocytes (WBCs). (F) The monocyte is the largest of the normal WBCs with a less dense nucleus and slate gray (or blue gray) cytoplasm. (G) The nucleus of the eosinophil is divided into two parts. (H) Fewer than one percent of circulating WBCs are basophils.

HOW BLOOD IS MADE

Blood cells form in the bone marrow. Most blood cells are made in the long bones, skull, pelvis, and sternum. Blood cells are also made in the liver, spleen, and in the yolk sac of a developing fetus.

Hematopoiesis is the process of blood cell production. Here's how it works. Young, immature cells in the bone marrow divide and differentiate. To *differentiate* means that cells take on different characteristics and begin to mature. These maturing cells become erythrocytes, leukocytes, and thrombocytes depending on what the body needs.

This process is influenced by many factors. Here are two important ones.

- The body's hormones affect the production of cells.
- Certain nutrients are required for the cells that are formed to function properly.

Once the cells reach maturity, they're released from the bone marrow and into the bloodstream. You'll read more about what each type of cell does and how that's related to hematology testing later in the chapter.

The Hematology Lab

The hematology lab analyzes blood cells, their quantities, and their characteristics to diagnose and manage many conditions. Some of the most common illnesses diagnosed in the hematology lab include:

- *Anemias.* **Anemias** are conditions resulting from reduced numbers of RBCs in the blood or from reductions in the amount of hemoglobin the RBCs contain.
- *Leukemias.* **Leukemias** are diseases in which unusually high numbers of abnormal WBCs are produced.
- *Infections.* These are invasions of the blood and body tissues by bacteria and other microorganisms. (A microorganism is a living thing that can only be seen under a microscope.)

Hematology also includes the study of **hemostasis.** This is the body's ability to keep blood in a fluid state in the vessels. The hematology lab helps evaluate patients who have trouble forming blood clots, as well as those who form clots unexpectedly in their blood vessels.

You'll encounter various units of measurement as you read this chapter. You can refer to the table below for an explanation of the prefixes in the metric system and their meanings. For example, you can see that *milli-* means "one-thousandth of." If something is a milliliter, you know it's one-thousandth of a liter. In hematology, the measurements you'll see the most are the ones that are less than the number 1, for example, *picogram.*

Prefixes of the Metric System

Decimal Multiples	Prefix	Symbol	Meaning
1,000,000,000,000	tera-	T	One trillion times
1,000,000,000	giga-	G	One billion times
1,000,000	mega-	M	One million times
1,000	kilo-	k	One thousand times
100	hector-	h	One hundred times
10	deka-	da	Ten times
1			One times
0.1	deci-	d	One-tenth of
0.01	centi-	c	One-hundredth of
0.001	milli-	m	One-thousandth of
0.000001	micro-	mu	One-millionth of
0.000000001	nano-	n	One-billionth of
0.000000000001	pico-	p	One-trillionth of
0.000000000000001	femto-	f	One-quadrillionth of

HEMATOLOGY TESTING

Hematology testing does more than just help diagnose and treat problems with the blood cells. It's also useful in detecting and dealing with the following types of problems:

- metabolic disorders—problems with the body's chemical and physical processes, such as growth and producing energy
- nutritional disorders—problems with how food is used for nourishment and body repair
- immunological disorders—problems resulting from bacteria, viruses, and other foreign substances in the body
- neoplastic disorders—problems related to abnormal growth of tissue, such as tumors

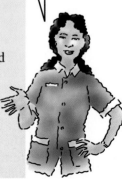

The word gigantic describes something that is really big, so it's no surprise that the prefix giga- means one billion times.

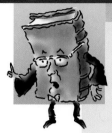

Legal Brief

HEMATOLOGY TESTS AND MEDICAL ASSISTANTS

Clinical Laboratory Improvement Amendments (CLIA) rules limit the tests medical assistants can perform to waived tests only. In general, medical assistants can't perform tests such as WBCs and RBCs if they involve the manual counting of cells. However, medical assistants who have extra training are allowed to perform some moderate-complexity tests.

Hematology tests medical assistants currently can perform include:

- erythrocyte sedimentation rate (not automated)
- hematocrit (all spun microhematocrit procedures)
- hemoglobin (selected methods)
- prothrombin time (selected methods)

The entire list of waived tests is updated regularly by the Centers for Medicare and Medicaid Services (CMS). As a medical assistant, you should know which tests you're allowed by law to perform.

Remember that even with waived tests, it's still possible to make a mistake. If test results are inaccurate, patients could go untreated or receive an improper diagnosis or treatment. In some cases, this could be disastrous.

To protect yourself and your employer against possible legal action, make sure you follow the proper procedures and the manufacturer's instructions for whatever test you are performing. Also, always stay within your scope of practice.

Complete Blood Count

The complete blood count (CBC), or hemogram, is one of the most frequently ordered lab tests. It consists of several related tests:

- WBC count and differential
- RBC count

- hemoglobin (Hgb) determination
- hematocrit (Hct) determination
- mean cell volume (MCV)
- mean corpuscular hemoglobin (MCH)
- mean corpuscular hemoglobin concentration (MCHC)
- platelet count

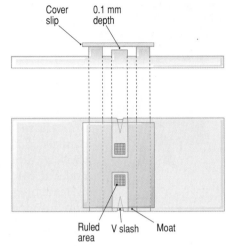

The Neubauer hemocytometer is an example of a manual counting chamber.

You'll read more about each of these tests later in this chapter.

A dilution of **whole blood** is prepared from a free-flowing finger puncture or from blood that has been anticoagulated (prevented from clotting) with EDTA (ethylenediaminetetraacetic acid). Whole blood is blood that has not been modified except for the addition of an anticoagulant. It is blood that has been taken directly from the body. The Hands On procedure on page 96 will show you how to prepare a whole blood dilution using the Unopette system.

Each kind of blood cell can then be counted using a manual counting chamber called a **hematocytometer** or a **hemocytometer.** However, automated cell counters have largely replaced the manual systems. There are many models of automated cell counters available, so that both the large laboratory and the smaller physician's office can use them.

WHITE BLOOD CELL COUNT AND DIFFERENTIAL

White blood cells (WBCs), or leukocytes, are the body's main line of defense against bacteria and viruses. Different types of WBCs have different functions in the body. Some circulate in the bloodstream. Others work their way into the body's tissues and cavities to do their job.

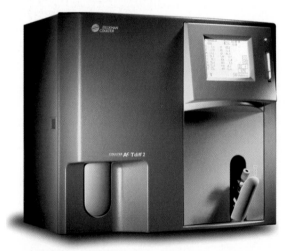

The COULTER A^c·T diff2 Hematology Analyzer is an example of an automated cell counter.

Closer Look   AUTOMATED BLOOD CELL COUNTERS

A number of companies have instruments that count and size blood cells. Each has its own specific way of doing it, but the basic method is the same. Here's how it works.

1. A whole blood sample (anticoagulated with EDTA) is taken in and diluted.

2. These dilutions are moved into counting chambers, where they are drawn through tiny holes, or apertures.

3. As the cells pass through the holes, an electrical current, a light beam, or a laser beam is interrupted.

4. The instrument counts each interruption as a cell. It can tell the size of the cell by the length of time the beam is interrupted or by the amount of light scatter.

Automated cell counters have become so highly developed that they can report a white blood cell differential accurately. They also measure hemoglobin, along with other tests, such as mean corpuscular hemoglobin (MCH). Their ability to measure such a wide variety of factors makes the complete blood count even more valuable.

    AEROSOL SAFETY

When handling blood specimens, you must take care to protect yourself from harm. In addition to avoiding direct contact with body fluids, you should also protect yourself from exposure to aerosols of blood. Aerosols are very fine droplets contained in a gas. In a lab, they can occur when blood tubes are opened.

How can you protect yourself? Besides wearing personal protective equipment (PPE), you can take steps to minimize the possibility of aerosols when opening blood collection tubes. Here are three ways to do this.

- Use special safety caps on blood collection tubes instead of the standard rubber tops. These caps don't

(continued)

AEROSOL SAFETY (continued)

allow aerosol when tubes are opened. The caps can be removed with one hand.

- When standard tops are already present on tubes, use a cap shield. These fit over the regular tops and prevent any aerosol or splash when the top is pulled out.

- If neither of these protective devices is available, cover the tube's standard rubber top with a folded paper towel before you remove it.

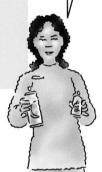

You might be familiar with aerosols as a mist sprayed out of a container of hair spray or air freshener.

The normal WBC range is 4,500–11,000/mm^3. A patient's WBC count can be figured using a hematocytometer counting chamber (manual) or an automated cell counter.

A WBC count measures the white blood cells in the **peripheral blood** (blood circulating in the body). The differential reveals the types of WBCs and the quantity of each. As you read earlier, the types of WBCs include:

- neutrophils
- lymphocytes
- monocytes
- eosinophils
- basophils

All types of WBCs are colorless. To study them, a blood sample must be smeared on a slide and then stained. This way, the different kinds of WBCs can be seen under a microscope. The Hands On procedure on page 100 shows how to make a peripheral blood smear. The Hands On

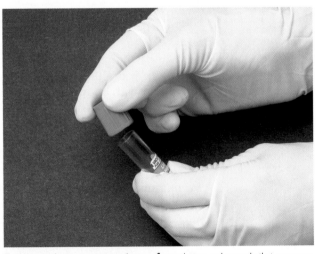

The Hemogard stopper protects the user from splatters and aerosols that can occur when a tube is uncapped.

procedure on page 102 explains how to stain a peripheral blood smear.

Once a blood sample has been stained, 100 WBCs are counted and divided according to type. Then, the different types are reported as percentages.

For more information on performing a WBC differential, see the Hands On procedure on page 103. CLIA rules don't allow medical assistants to perform WBC differentials. However, they are permitted to prepare and stain the samples from which manual differentials are done. Therefore, it's useful to learn the testing technique so that you can make sure the slides you prepare are usable.

Neutrophils

Neutrophils are the most plentiful leukocytes (WBCs) and the main granulocyte. Here's how they move in the blood.

1. Neutrophils are released from the bone marrow.
2. They circulate in the blood for about seven hours.
3. Then, they move into the tissues where they can perform their function.

Closer Look   LEUKOPENIA AND LEUKOCYTOSIS

Leukopenia is a condition when there are too few WBCs in the body. Several factors can decrease the number of WBCs. Here are some of the more common ones:

- chemical toxicity
- poor nutrition
- chronic or overwhelming infection
- certain malignancies

Too many WBCs result in a condition called leukocytosis. Among the things that can cause it are:

- infection
- inflammatory condition
- certain drugs
- injury to tissue
- certain malignancies

Neutrophils defend the body against bacteria by phagocytosis, or surrounding and digesting them. The bacteria are killed by digestive **enzymes.** An enzyme is a protein that starts a chemical reaction. Eventually, the digestive enzymes kill the neutrophil, too.

Normally about 50 to 70 percent of WBCs are neutrophils. The percentage is higher in patients who have bacterial infections.

When a neutrophil is stained, it has a light pink cytoplasm. The nucleus is dark purple and usually has five or fewer segments. If a patient's neutrophils have more than five segments (hypersegmented), this condition can mean a vitamin B_{12} or **folate** deficiency. (Folate is an essential nutrient.)

A band (or stab) is a younger version of the neutrophil, not fully mature. Its appearance is much the same as a regular neutrophil, but its nucleus isn't segmented. The normal percentage of bands is zero to five percent. A higher percentage may indicate acute infections that require immediate attention

- Neutrophilia (an increase in neutrophils) can be a sign of inflammation or some bacterial infections, such as syphilis and tuberculosis.

- Neutropenia (a low number of neutrophils) can result after an overwhelming infection or after certain drugs have been given to a patient.

Ask the Professional   TEST CONFIDENTIALITY

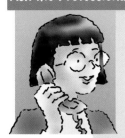

Q: *Yesterday, I called a patient to remind her about her office appointment. I also wanted to remind her to get her T cell count drawn at the lab before coming in. I left that message with the person who answered the phone. When the patient arrived for her appointment, she was upset that I had mentioned the name of the test in the message. I don't understand. I didn't give out any test results or disclose any information about her condition. Did I do something wrong?*

A: Yes, you did. Not only are a patient's test results confidential, but the kind of test is, too. You violated the patient's privacy when you revealed the reason for the lab visit. In this case, a T cell count is an AIDS indicator, which is highly sensitive information. In such situations, you should leave a message reminding a patient to go to the lab, but you can't tell why she's to go there.

Lymphocytes

Lymphocytes are the next most common leukocyte. They're also the smallest. A lymphocyte's purpose is to recognize that a foreign cell or particle is a threat to the body and then make antibodies to destroy it. These antibodies coat the foreign cell or particle, and then one of two things happens.

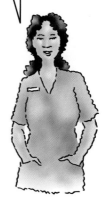

The five types of white blood cells (WBCs), or leukocytes, in order of their abundance are neutrophils, lymphocytes, monocytes, eosinophils, and basophils.

- The pathogen is destroyed by being surrounded and digested (the phagocytic system); or
- A group of chemicals in the blood destroys the foreign cell or particle by puncturing holes in its membranes (the complement system).

The normal percentage of lymphocytes is 20 to 40 percent. That number is higher, however, in patients with viral infections, such as infectious mononucleosis.

Most lymphocytes live four to seven days, although some can last years or decades. When lymphocytes are stained, they have a small, round, dark purple nucleus, and their cytoplasm is sky blue.

Monocytes

Monocytes are the third most common leukocyte. They're twice the size of nonreactive lymphocytes and slightly larger than neutrophils. The main purpose of monocytes is to digest foreign cells or particles—much like neutrophils—and to assist the lymphocytes in the destruction of foreign cells or particles by antibodies.

The shape of a monocyte's nucleus can vary. When a monocyte is stained, the cytoplasm is gray-blue and looks like ground glass.

Monocytes stay in the bloodstream for about three days and then move into body tissues. The normal percentage of monocytes is three to eight percent.

Eosinophils and Basophils

Eosinophils are the fourth most common leukocyte. Their function in the body is not completely understood. The nucleus of an eosinophil is divided into two segments, with large orange granules in the cytoplasm. The normal percentage of eosinophils is zero to six percent, but it's higher in allergic reactions and some infections, especially parasitic ones.

Basophils are the least plentiful type of leukocyte. In fact, fewer than one percent of WBCs are basophils. The nucleus of a basophil is either two or three segments. When stained, very large dark blue-purple granules appear in the cytoplasm.

See the table below for a review of these WBCs.

Types and Charactersics of WBCs

Cell	Percent of Normal WBC	Size (microns)	Size Relative to the Diameter of an RBC (7 microns)	Function	Nucleus
Lymphocytes (Lymph)	20–40%	10	X 1.25	Fight viral infections	Dark purple; normal RBCs are the same size as nucleus of lymph
Reactive lymphocytes	0–5%	10–20	X 2 to 3	Usually B lymphocytes producing antibodies to fight infections	Nucleus not as dark as regular lymph; usually smooth consistency
Segmented neutrophils (Segs)	50–70%	12–15	X 2	Fight bacterial infections	Dark purple; 2–5 lobes
Neutrophilic band (Band)	0–5%	12–15	X 2	An immature Seg; a young warrior that doesn't fight infections as well as a Seg	Dark purple; tube-shaped, may be twisted and turned, but not pinched
Eosinophils (Eos)	0–6%	12–15	X 2	Slightly increased in allergic reactions 10–15%; markedly increased in parasitic	Dark purple; 2–3 lobes, usually obscured by orange granules

Types and Charactersics of WBCs (*continued*)

Cell	Percent of Normal WBC	Size (microns)	Size Relative to the Diameter of an RBC (7 microns)	Function	Nucleus
				infections, up to 40% of WBC	
Basophils (Baso)	0–1%	12–15	X 2	Granules contain histamine and heparin	Dark purple; 2–5 lobes, usually obscured by purple granules
Monocytes (Mono)	3–8%	18–23	X 2.5 to 3.5	Clean up cell and microbe debris; the "garbage collector" after the battle	Lighter purple to blue; less dense

RED BLOOD CELL COUNT

Red blood cells (RBCs), or erythrocytes, transport gases between the lungs and the body tissues. They are shaped like disks that are concave on both sides and contain hemoglobin. Their special design allows them to easily change shape and pass through small capillaries. They exchange gases in the body tissues and lungs. Here's how that works.

1. Blood moves through the capillary bed of the lungs. The RBCs release carbon dioxide that was picked up at the tissues. Then, the RBCs bind oxygen.

2. As the blood leaves the lungs and circulates to the organs, oxygen is released from the RBCs into the tissues. At the same time, carbon dioxide (the byproduct of metabolism) goes into the blood and is brought back to the lungs to be exhaled.

Red Blood Cell Production

RBCs are made in the bone marrow with all the other blood cells. The hormone **erythropoietin** is released from the kidneys and influences the production of RBCs. This is a reason why individuals with kidney problems may become anemic.

Erythropoietin stimulates the production of RBCs to increase blood oxygen levels. Here's what happens.

- When the body detects **hypoxia** (inadequate oxygen reaching the body's tissues), erythropoietin travels to the bone marrow to increase RBC production.
- The increase in RBCs corrects the anemia by releasing more RBCs into circulation in the body.

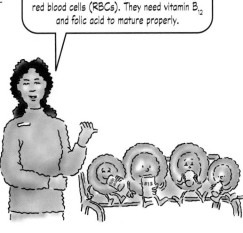

Nutrition can affect the quality and quantity of red blood cells (RBCs). They need vitamin B$_{12}$ and folic acid to mature properly.

At first, RBCs have a nucleus. As they mature, the nucleus is pushed out. The color of their cytoplasm changes from blue to red. A mature RBC is a pale red biconcave (concave on both sides) disk that is able to squeeze through very small capillaries. The average RBC lives about 120 days.

Measuring Red Blood Cells

Measuring RBCs helps to detect anemia, which can be caused by:

- decreased RBC production (as in iron deficiency)
- increased RBC destruction (as in **hemolytic anemia**)
- blood loss

The normal range of RBCs differs among men and women. For men, the normal range is 4.6 to 6.2 million/mm^3. For women, the range is 4.2 to 5.4 million/mm^3.

A report on the **morphology,** or appearance, of RBCs is included in a WBC differential count. The report comments on variations in the size **(anisocytosis)** and shape **(poikilocytosis)** of the RBCs. The table below describes some common RBC abnormalities and the conditions they may indicate.

Erythrocyte (Red Blood Cell) Abnormalities

Abnormality	Associated Conditions
Hypochromasia—reduced hemoglobin in RBCs; appear lighter with more area of central pallor	Anemias (especially iron deficiency), **thalassemia** (a hemolytic anemia)
Hyperchromasia—increased hemoglobin in RBCs; appear to have less or no area of central pallor	**Megaloblastic anemia** (characterized by large, dysfunctional RBCs), hereditary **spherocytosis** (condition in which nearly all the RBCs are spherocytes)

Erythrocyte (Red Blood Cell) Abnormalities (*continued*)

Abnormality	Associated Conditions
Polychromasia—some RBCs have a blue color	Hemolysis, acute blood loss
Microcytosis—RBCs are smaller than usual	Iron deficiency anemia, thalassemia
Macrocytosis—RBCs are larger than normal	B_{12} and folate deficiencies, megaloblastic anemias
Elliptocytes/ovalocytes—RBCs are distinctly oval in shape	Hereditary **elliptocytosis** (condition in which all or almost all of the RBCs are elliptical or oval in shape), iron deficiency anemia, **myelofibrosis** (disorder in which bone marrow tissue develops in abnormal sites), **sickle cell anemia** (hereditary anemia characterized by the presence of sickle-shaped RBCs)
Target cells—RBCs resemble targets with light and dark rings	Liver impairment, anemias (especially thalassemia), **hemoglobin C disease** (genetic blood disorder)
Schistocytes—RBCs are fragmented	Hemolysis, burns, **intravascular coagulation** (clot formation within the vessels)
Spherocytes—RBCs show no area of central paleness	Hereditary spherocytosis, hemolytic anemias, burns
Burr cells—RBCs have small, regular spicules (sharp points)	Artifact as blood dries, **hyperosmolarity** (a condition of increased numbers of dissolved substances in the plasma)

Hematocrit Testing. The percentage of RBCs in whole blood is called the hematocrit. For example, if a patient has a hematocrit of 40, it means that 40 percent of the patient's total blood volume is RBCs. The other 60 percent is plasma.

The purpose of the hematocrit test is to detect anemia. To get a hematocrit measurement, the blood is centrifuged to pack the RBCs into one area so a percentage can be read. A microhematocrit centrifuge doesn't actually calculate the hematocrit. Instead, it must be read on a machine or chart. Cell counting machines measure the RBC count and the mean cell volume (MCV) and then calculate the hematocrit from these two values using the formula for MCV. The normal hematocrit range for men is 45 to 52. For women, it's 37 to 48. For guidance on performing a hematocrit test, see the Hands On procedure on page 104.

Mean Corpuscular Volume. The mean corpuscular volume (MCV) test measures the average size of a patient's RBCs. The normal range for MCV is 80 to 95 **femtoliters** (fL). (A femtoliter is equal to one-quadrillionth of a liter.) Knowing the MCV helps to diagnose anemias, such as those caused by the nutritional deficiencies that affect RBC production.

Too little iron often results in microcytosis (when the MCV is below 80 fL). This test finding, along with RBC counts, hematocrit and hemoglobin tests, and tests for forms of iron and related compounds, may lead to a diagnosis of iron deficiency anemia.

A deficiency of vitamin B_{12} or folic acid is often the cause of macrocytosis (when the MCV is above 95 fL). This abnormality can also indicate anemia. In addition, liver disorders can raise the MCV.

Erythrocyte Sedimentation Rate. Erythrocyte sedimentation rate (ESR or sed rate) measures the rate at which RBCs settle out in a tube. Here's the basic process for measuring the ESR.

1. Place anticoagulated blood in a calibrated glass tube.
2. Allow blood to settle undisturbed for one hour.
3. At the end of the hour, measure the distance in millimeters that the RBCs have fallen.

The normal range for ESR in men is 0 to 10 mm/hour. For women, it's 0 to 20 mm/hour. A higher ESR value doesn't point to a specific disorder, but it does indicate inflammation or other conditions that indicate increased or altered proteins in the blood (for example, rheumatoid arthritis). The ESR can also be higher in patients who are pregnant or who have an infection. The more quickly the RBCs fall in the tube, the greater the inflammation is in the patient.

The Hands On procedure on page 106 provides detailed steps for performing a Westergren ESR. Currently, CLIA rules permit medical assistants to perform only manual ESR tests. However, automated ESR tests are available and they may soon become waived tests. In an automated ESR, a centrifuge spins the

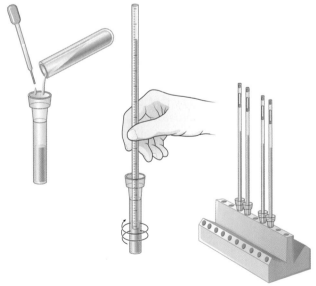

Westergren Dispette System for ESR determination. Left: After mixing four parts EDTA-anticoagulated whole blood with one part 0.85-percent saline, the mixture is poured into a vial. Center: Dispette is placed in vial using a twisting motion until blood reaches bottom of safety autozeroing plug. Right: Vial and Dispette are placed upright in a special rack for 60 minutes before reading the ESR.

sample for three minutes, forcing the RBCs to the end of the tube. About 100 measurements are taken during the process. The ESR is calculated from these measurements.

Measuring Hemoglobin

Hemoglobin is the part of the red blood cell that binds the gases it carries. There are millions of hemoglobin molecules in each RBC.

Each hemoglobin molecule also contains four protein chains called globins. The most common globin chains are named alpha and beta. Newborns have some gamma (fetal) globin chains instead of alpha chains in their fetal hemoglobin. Fetal hemoglobin percentages should drop to less than three percent after six months. When there's a defect in those globin chains, patients have abnormal hemoglobins. For example, sickle cell anemia is one condition caused by abnormal hemoglobins.

Like RBCs in general, the normal range for hemoglobin differs among men and women. For men, the normal range is 13 to 18 g/dL. For women, it's 12 to 16 g/dL. Anemia can be detected with a hemoglobin measurement—this shows the body's ability to oxygenate tissues.

MORE RED BLOOD CELL INDICES

The purpose of the mean corpuscular hemoglobin (MCH) and the mean corpuscular hemoglobin concentration (MCHC) is to show the relative hemoglobin concentration in the blood. Both the MCH and the MCHC must be calculated. When RBCs don't have enough hemoglobin, they're called hypochromic.

The MCH represents the average weight of hemoglobin molecules in a single RBC. The normal range is 27 to 31 **picograms.** A picogram is one-trillionth of a gram. The MCHC represents the density of the hemoglobin molecule in a single RBC. The normal range is 32 to 36 g/dL. Certain conditions can cause an increase or decrease of the MCH or the MCHC.

PLATELET COUNT

Like other blood cells, platelets, or thrombocytes, are made in the bone marrow. Platelets are not actually cells, but cell fragments. They can attach themselves to damaged endothelium (a layer of flattened cells that lines the inside of some body cavities). Platelets perform two important functions.

- They aid in sealing wounds and stopping bleeding until a clot can form.
- They help initiate the clotting factors to form a sturdier fibrin clot.

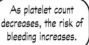

As platelet count decreases, the risk of bleeding increases.

The normal number of platelets ranges from 150,000 to 450,000/mm³. Having too few platelets is called thrombocytopenia. This can be caused by a variety of conditions. Increased bleeding also can result when the number of platelets is decreased.

Having too many platelets is called thrombocytosis. This condition is often benign. It's sometimes seen after a splenectomy or during an inflammatory disease. However, marked thrombocytosis (above 1 million/mm³) may be associated with increased clotting, or even severe bleeding if the platelets aren't functioning properly.

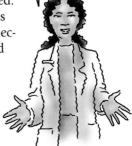

Platelets are much smaller than RBCs. When stained, they are a light purplish blue. They have an irregular shape and no nucleus.

Coagulation Tests

Coagulation tests measure the ability of whole blood to form a clot. When the body suffers a cut, proteins in the blood, called clotting factors, work together to form a clot. Here's how the whole process happens.

1. *Vasoconstriction.* The vein narrows to reduce blood loss.
2. *Platelet plug forms.* Platelets stick to the wound and form a plug to slow or stop the blood flow.
3. *Fibrin clot forms.* The blood's clotting factors form a clot at the site of the wound.
4. *Clotlysis and vascular repair.* As the body repairs the damage (the cut heals), another set of proteins slowly dissolves the clot.

The two most common tests for determining how well a fibrin clot can form are prothrombin time (PT) and partial thromboplastin time (PTT).

These tests are common when treating patients with clotting problems (including heart attacks, stroke, and pulmonary embolism). When treating these patients, the physician may start patients on two medications.

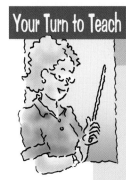

Your Turn to Teach

HELPING PATIENTS UNDERSTAND THROMBOCYTOPENIA

Patients with low platelet counts may need instruction to help them understand their condition and the precautions they should take.

Tell patients that if they bruise easily, any of these other signs could indicate thrombocytopenia:

- prolonged bleeding from a cut
- tiny red or purple spots on the skin (called petechiae)
- black or bloody stool
- brown or red urine
- nose bleeds or bleeding gums
- increased vaginal bleeding

Instruct patients with low platelet counts to take these precautions:

- Avoid aspirin or any medication that contains aspirin. If you aren't sure if a medication is safe, talk to the physician before taking it.
- Use a soft toothbrush. Brush gently and floss carefully.
- Use an electric shaver instead of a razor.
- Avoid foods that might irritate your digestive tract or make you constipated.
- Avoid clothing with tight-fitting elastic waist or wristbands. Always wear shoes.
- Avoid enemas, rectal thermometers, and suppositories. Women should avoid douches and tampons.
- Blow your nose gently.

Advise patients with thrombocytopenia to ask the doctor if sexual intercourse is a safe activity. Also, tell them to call the office right away in the following situations:

- new bruising or petechiae
- bleeding from your nose, mouth, or gums
- blood in your urine or stool
- a headache that doesn't go away

- Heparin is used for immediate inhibition of the formation of new clots.
- Coumadin is used for the long-term inhibition of new clot formation.

PROTHROMBIN TIME

The prothrombin time (PT) is a test designed to measure clotting time. It is used to monitor Coumadin therapy. Here's how it works.

- Calcium and **thromboplastin** (a substance that starts the clotting process) are added to the patient's plasma.
- The clotting time is then observed. The normal range is 12 to 15 seconds, but your lab may set its own range.

The following factors may lengthen a patient's PT:

- liver disease
- vitamin K deficiency
- Coumadin (oral anticoagulant) therapy

When the PT starts to show abnormal results, it's a sign that the physician needs to adjust the heparin and Coumadin therapy. There are several point-of-care instruments that medical assistants can use in the medical office to determine PT times.

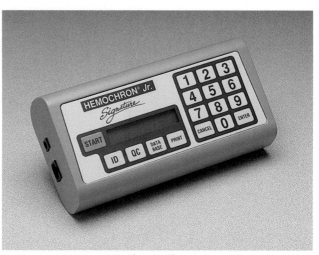

The Hemochron Jr. is an example of a point-of-care instrument that can be used in the medical office to determine PT times.

PARTIAL THROMBOPLASTIN TIME

The partial thromboplastin time (PTT) is a two-stage test to determine clotting time. Here's how it works.

- Partially activated thromboplastin is incubated with the patient's plasma.
- Next, calcium is added.
- Then, the clotting time is figured. The normal range is 32 to 51 seconds, but like a PT test, a lab sets its own range.

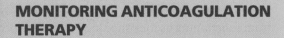

Running Smoothly

MONITORING ANTICOAGULATION THERAPY

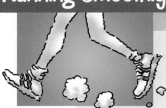

What if a patient doesn't cooperate with taking a PT test?

A patient has been taking Coumadin and is supposed to come in for a PT test. However, the patient never shows up for his appointment. What should you do?

First, let the physician know. It's the physician's responsibility to decide whether a refill should be called in to the pharmacy. Then, try to contact the patient to find out why he didn't return for the blood work. Perhaps transportation is a problem. Many communities have programs where health care workers will draw patients' blood in their homes.

- Make sure the patient understands the purpose of the medication and why the blood tests are important to his health.

- Inform the patient about the dangers of self-dosing Coumadin. For example, he could experience excessive bleeding with an overdose and clotting with an underdose.

- Document all phone conversations with the patient, including the date, time, and message. Also, record the patient's responses.

> When documenting a patient's response, try to quote his exact words when possible. This provides the most accurate information on patient communication.

PTT can be delayed when certain clotting factor deficiencies are present in the blood, especially ones that cause hemophilia (uncontrolled bleeding). Heparin (anticoagulant) therapy also prolongs the PTT. This is why the PTT test is often used to monitor heparin therapy.

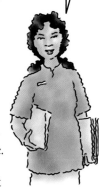

BLEEDING TIME

The purpose of the bleeding time test is to determine the time required for the blood to stop flowing from a very small wound.

To conduct the test, an incision one millimeter deep is made on the inside of the forearm with an automated cutting device.

Normal bleeding times range from two to six minutes. Longer-than-normal bleeding times can occur when platelet numbers are low or when platelet function isn't normal. Aspirin or other anti-inflammatory medications can also keep platelets from functioning as they should. Other very specific bleeding disorders can affect bleeding time.

Bleeding times may be measured before surgery when the patient's family history includes increased bruising or bleeding. More often, a lab test to evaluate platelet function is done instead. This has made the need for bleeding times less necessary.

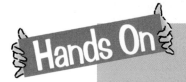

Hands On

PREPARING A WHOLE BLOOD DILUTION USING THE UNOPETTE SYSTEM   3-1

To prepare a whole blood dilution using the Unopette system, you'll need the following equipment: Unopette system and gauze.

Follow these steps to prepare a whole blood dilution using the Unopette system:

1. Wash your hands.

2. Get your equipment ready. Put on gloves.

3. Pierce the diaphragm in the neck of the plastic reservoir.
   - Push the tip of the shield on the capillary pipette though the diaphragm.
   - When you insert the shield, use a twisting motion.
   - Then, remove the outer protective shield from the pipette.

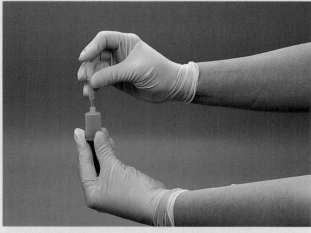

Make sure you push the shield through the diaphragm firmly.

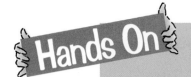

PREPARING A WHOLE BLOOD DILUTION USING THE UNOPETTE SYSTEM (*continued*)   **3-1**

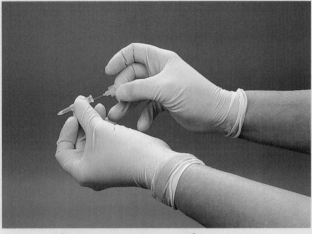

Remove the outer protective shield from the pipette.

4. Fill the pipette with free-flowing whole blood.
   - You may get the blood by performing a skin puncture or from a well-mixed lavender top tube specimen.
   - If filling from a tube, place the tip of the Unopette just below the surface of the blood. Allow capillary action to fill the tube completely.

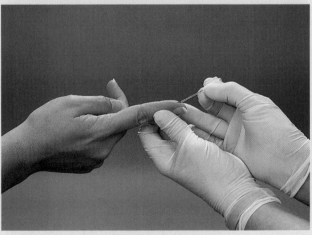

Draw the sample into the pipette from free-flowing skin puncture or tube.

(*continued*)

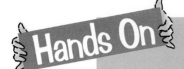

Hands On

PREPARING A WHOLE BLOOD DILUTION USING THE UNOPETTE SYSTEM (*continued*)   3-1

5. Wipe the pipette with gauze or lab tissue to remove excess blood, but be careful not to wipe across the pipette's tip. This is because the gauze could absorb some of the blood sample and cause false test results.

6. Gently squeeze the reservoir to help expel some of the air. Make sure you don't push out any of the diluting fluids. Getting some of the air out of the reservoir will help create a vacuum that will help when filling the unit.

7. Cover the opposite end of the pipette from where the blood came in with your finger. Keeping pressure on the sides of the reservoir, insert the pipette through the hole previously made in the diaphragm until the lower collar on the pipette makes a seal with the neck on the reservoir.

8. Once you have achieved a seal, remove your finger from the end of the pipette and simultaneously release the pressure exerted on the sides of the reservoir.

9. Gently squeeze and release the reservoir several times to force the diluting fluids just slightly into but not out of the pipette's overflow chamber.

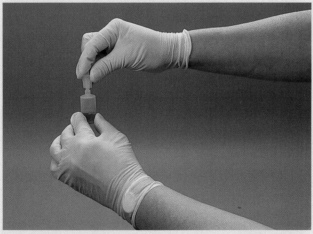

Squeeze the reservoir slightly to force out some air. When you release your squeeze on the reservoir in the next step, the vacuum will draw your sample into the reservoir.

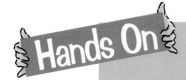
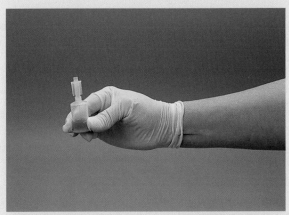

Gently squeezing and releasing the reservoir several times helps to rinse blood from the pipette and ensure proper dilution. Don't squeeze the reservoir hard enough to expel fluid.

10. Put your index finger over the opening of the pipette's over-flow chamber and gently turn it upside down or swirl the container several times to mix. Remove the pipette, invert it, and insert it back into the neck of the reservoir with the pipette sticking out. Next, cover the pipette with the plastic protective cover removed earlier. You can place the whole reservoir-pipette assembly on a blood rocker, if one is available.

11. Carefully label the specimen with all the required information.

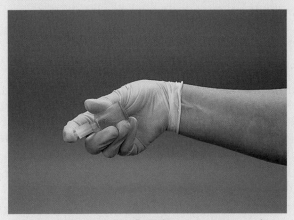

Although the specimen must be well-mixed to get accurate test results, you must mix it gently to avoid destroying cells.

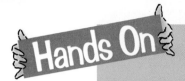

MAKING A PERIPHERAL BLOOD SMEAR

3-2

To prepare a peripheral blood smear, you'll need the following equipment: clean glass slides with frosted ends, a pencil, a well-mixed whole blood specimen, and a transfer pipette.

Follow these steps to prepare a blood sample for microscopic examination:

1. Wash your hands.
2. Get your equipment ready.
3. Greet and identify the patient. Explain the procedure. Ask for and answer any questions.
4. Put on gloves, an impervious gown, and a face shield.
5. Perform a venipuncture as described in Chapter 2 to get an EDTA (lavender-top tube) blood specimen from your patient.
6. Label the slide with the patient's name or identification number on the frosted area using a pencil.
7. Hold the slide flat between the thumb and first finger on your non-dominant hand. Place a drop of blood 1 cm from the frosting at one end of the slide. The slide also can be held on a flat surface and the smear made on the surface. Try both ways and see which is more comfortable and gets the best results.
8. Use your thumb and forefinger on your dominant hand to hold the second (spreader) slide against the surface of the first slide at a 30-degree angle.
   - The angle of the spreader slide may have to be greater for large or thin drops of blood.
   - The angle of the spreader slide may have to be less than 30 degrees for small or thick drops.
   Move the spreader slide back until it is touching the drop of blood. Allow the blood to spread under the edge for a fraction of a second. Then push the spreader slide at a medium speed toward the other end of the slide. Make sure the two slides are in contact the entire time.
9. Allow the slide to air dry. (The photograph shows properly and improperly prepared smears.)
10. Properly take care of or dispose of equipment and supplies. Clean your work area. Then, remove your gloves, gown, and face shield, and wash your hands.

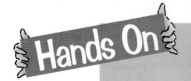
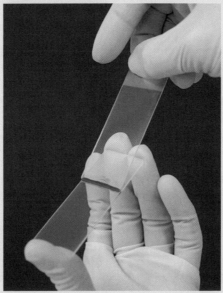

Make sure you don't hesitate too long before pushing the
spreader slide toward the other end of the slide. If you wait too
long, platelets will collect along the edge of the spreader slide.

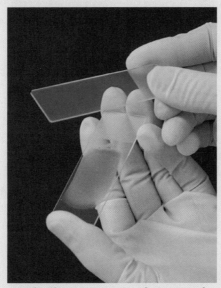

A thin film of blood is desired at the feathered end of
the smear. After staining, a proper smear should have
a significant area where the RBCs are close to each
other, but not on top of each other. Too much blood on
the slide will make the smear unusable.

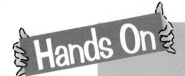

STAINING A PERIPHERAL BLOOD SMEAR

3-3

To stain a peripheral blood smear, you'll need the following equipment: a staining rack, Wright's stain, Giemsa stain, a prepared slide, and tweezers.

Follow these steps to stain a peripheral blood smear:

1. Wash your hands.

2. Get your equipment ready.

3. Put on gloves, an impervious gown, and a face shield.

4. Get the dried blood smear. Keep in mind that a smear made from blood that's more that four hours old may have deteriorated cells.

5. Place the slide on a stain rack, blood side up. Then, flood the slide with Wright's stain. Leave the stain on the slide for three to five minutes or for the time specified by the manufacturer. The alcohol in Wright's stain helps fix the blood to the slide.

6. Use your tweezers to tilt the slide so that the stain drains off. Then, apply equal amounts of Giemsa stain and water or a Wright's buffer. A green sheen will appear on the slide's surface. Let the solution remain on the slide for five minutes or the time specified by the manufacturer. This helps improve the quality of the stain.

7. Again, hold the slide with your tweezers. Gently rinse the slide with water to remove any excess stain. Wipe off the back of the slide with gauze. Stand the slide upright and allow it to dry.

8. Properly take care of or dispose of equipment and supplies. Clean your work area. Then, remove your gloves, gown, and face shield, and wash your hands.

Note: Some manufacturers provide a simple method that consists of dipping the smear in a staining solution, then water, and then rinsing. Directions provided by the manufacturer vary with the specific staining system.

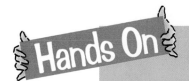
To perform a white blood cell differential, you'll need the following equipment: a stained peripheral blood smear, a microscope, immersion oil, paper, and a recording tabulator (differential calculator).

Follow these steps to perform a WBC differential:

1. Wash your hands.

2. Get your equipment ready.

3. Put the stained slide on the microscope. Focus on the feathered edge of the smear and scan with the low-power objective to make sure the cells are evenly distributed and properly stained.

4. Carefully turn the nosepiece to the high-power objective and bring the slide into focus using the fine adjustment.

5. Carefully turn the nosepiece so the point of focus on the slide is between the high-power objective and the oil objective.

6. Place a drop of oil on the slide and move the oil immersion lens into place using the fine adjustment. Focus and begin to identify any leukocytes. (The oil helps to provide a path for the light between the specimen on the slide and the oil immersion objective.)

7. Record on a tally sheet or differential counter the types of white cells you find. This way, you'll be able to calculate accurate percentages.

8. Move the stage so the next field is in view. Identify any white cells in this field and then continue to the next field. The goal is to view as many fields as necessary to count 100 white cells. Move the stage systematically so you know where you counted and where you still need to count, to find new cells, and to avoid counting the same cell twice.

9. Record the number of each type of leukocyte (WBC) as a percentage. Remember that because you counted 100 cells, each cell represents one percentage point.

10. Properly take care of or dispose of equipment and supplies. Clean your work area. Then, remove your gloves and wash your hands.

Note: A trained laboratory technologist is the one who performs a WBC differential. Abnormal cells can appear in peripheral blood and the technologist must have specific training to recognize them. A platelet estimation, RBC morphology, and platelet morphology are done while doing a differential.

Hands On

PERFORMING A MANUAL MICROHEMATOCRIT DETERMINATION

3-5

To perform a manual microhematocrit determination, you'll need the following equipment: microcollection tubes, sealing clay, a microhematocrit centrifuge, and a microhematocrit-reading device:

Follow these steps to perform a manual microhematocrit determination:

1. Wash your hands.

2. Get your equipment ready.

3. Put on gloves, a gown, and a face shield.

4. Use one of the following methods to draw blood into the capillary tube.

   A. *Directly from a capillary puncture:*
   - Touch the tip of the capillary tube to the blood at the wound and allow the tube to fill to three-quarters or the indicated mark.
   - For a finger stick, use heparinized capillary tubes.
   - Place your forefinger over the top of the capillary tube, wipe excess blood off its sides, and push its bottom into the sealing clay. (Make sure you push the end opposite to the end the blood was drawn in.) Use caution while sealing tubes as they can break and puncture gloves and skin if you use too much force.
   - Then, draw a second specimen in the same way. (The second tube is for a duplicate test as a part of quality control.)

   B. *From a well-mixed EDTA tube of whole blood:*
   - Touch the tip of the capillary tube to the blood in the EDTA tube and allow the capillary tube to fill three-quarters.
   - Place your forefinger over the top of the capillary tube, wipe excess blood off its sides, and push its bottom into the sealing clay. (Make sure you push the end opposite to the end the blood was drawn in.) Use caution while sealing tubes as they can break and puncture gloves and skin if you use too much force.
   - Draw a second specimen in the same way. (The second tube is for a duplicate test as a part of quality control.)

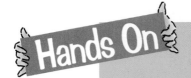

PERFORMING A MANUAL MICROHEMATOCRIT DETERMINATION (*continued*)

3-5

5. Place the tubes, with the clay-sealed end out, in the radial grooves of the microhematocrit centrifuge opposite each other. Put the lid on the grooved area and tighten by turning the knob clockwise. Close the lid. Spin for five minutes or as directed by the manufacturer.

6. Remove the tubes from the centrifuge and read the results. Instructions on how to do this are printed on the device. Take the average and report it as a percentage. (The figure shows the determinations of microhematocrit values. Results should be within two percent of each other. Results that have greater than a two-percent variation are unreliable. A three-percent difference is the equivalent of a patient losing about a pint of blood.)

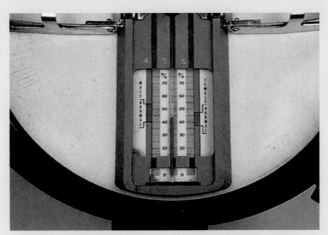

Note how the results are displayed on this centrifuge-reading device.

7. Dispose of the microhematocrit tubes in a biohazard container. Properly take care of or dispose of other equipment and supplies. Clean your work area. Then, remove your gloves, gown, and face shield, and wash your hands.

Note: Some microhematocrit centrifuges have the scale printed in the machine at the radial grooves.

Hands On

PERFORMING A WESTERGREN ERYTHROCYTE SEDIMENTATION RATE

To use the Westergren method for finding the erythrocyte sedimentation rate (ESR), you'll need the following equipment: a whole blood sample collected in EDTA (free of clots and less than four hours old), a Sediplast system vial prefilled with 0.2 mL of 3.8 percent sodium citrate, an autozero calibrated Sediplast pipette, a sedrate rack, and a disposable transfer pipette.

Follow these steps to determine the ESR:

1. Wash your hands.

2. Get your equipment ready.

3. Put on gloves and personal protective equipment.

4. Remove the stopper on the prefilled vial. Using a transfer pipette, fill the vial to the bottom of the indicated fill line with 0.8 mL of blood to make the required 4:1 dilution. (The test can also be run with no dilution.)

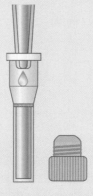

Use a transfer pipette to fill the vial.

5. Replace the pierceable stopper and gently invert several times. This way, there will be a good mixture of blood and diluent.

6. Place the vial in its rack on a level surface. Carefully insert the pipette through the pierceable stopper using a rotating downward pressure until the pipette comes in contact with the bottom of the vial. The pipette will autozero the blood and any excess will flow into the reservoir compartment.

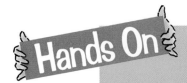

3-6

PERFORMING A WESTERGREN ERYTHROCYTE SEDIMENTATION RATE (*continued*)

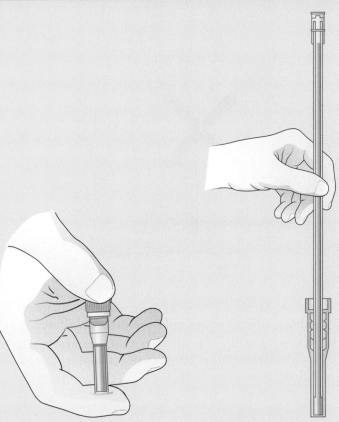

Invert the vial to get a good mixture of blood and diluent.

Insert the pipette through the stopper.

7. Make sure the pipette makes firm contact with the bottom of the vial. Otherwise, you may get inaccurate test results.

8. Let the sample stand for exactly one hour and then read the numerical results of the erythrocyte sedimentation in millimeters. Make sure the test is set up on a surface that is free from vibration and away from anything that may cause a change in temperature (windows, refrigerators,

(*continued*)

Hands On

PERFORMING A WESTERGREN ERYTHROCYTE SEDIMENTATION RATE (*continued*)

3-6

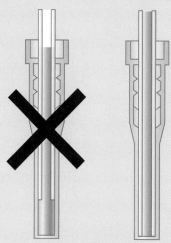

It's essential that the pipette makes firm contact with the bottom of the vial.

motors, AC ducts). Most of these will cause an increase in sedimentation rate, but cold will cause a decrease.

9. Properly take care of or dispose of equipment and supplies. Clean your work area. Then remove your gloves and other PPE and wash your hands.

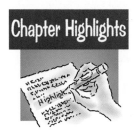

Chapter Highlights

- There are three basic types of blood cells—erythrocytes, leukocytes, and thrombocytes.
- Blood tests can help diagnose anemias and infections.
- Medical assistants perform a variety of important duties in hematological testing.
- Several types of blood tests are CLIA waived, which means the medical assistant can perform these tests in a typical physician office setting.
- The most common hematological tests are the complete blood count (CBC), erythrocyte sedimentation rate (ESR or sed rate), and coagulation tests.
- Red blood cells (RBCs), or erythrocytes, transport gases (mainly oxygen and carbon dioxide) between the lungs and the body tissues.
- The mean cell volume measures the average size of the RBCs.
- The purpose of the mean corpuscular hemoglobin (MCH) and the mean corpuscular hemoglobin concentration (MCHC) is to show the relative hemoglobin concentration in a single RBC.
- Coagulation tests such as prothrombin time (PT) and partial thromboplastin time (PTT) help to determine the patient's ability to maintain hemostasis.

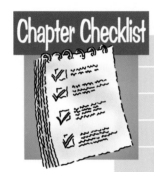

Chapter 4

IMMUNOLOGY AND IMMUNOHEMATOLOGY

Chapter Checklist

- Describe the different types of immunity
- Identify the different types of antibodies
- List the reasons for immunological testing
- Describe the antigen-antibody reaction
- Explain the principles of agglutination testing and ELISA
- Summarize the proper storage and handling of immunology test kits
- Describe the ways that quality control is applied to immunology testing
- List and describe immunology tests most commonly performed in the medical office or physician office lab
- Perform an HCG pregnancy test
- Perform a Group A Rapid Strep Test
- Identify the major blood types and explain why differences in blood type exist
- Describe how blood is typed and explain why this testing is important

Immunology is the study of how the body distinguishes between self and non-self, and how the body works to eliminate infectious agents. After reading this chapter, you'll better understand how your body remains strong and healthy. You'll also learn about immunology testing in this chapter and why it is used to test for certain conditions. As many immunology tests are performed in physician office lab (POL), you will need to learn how to perform them to achieve accurate results.

Immunology Basics

If you're studying immunology in a lab, you'll be looking at or for antigens and antibodies.

Antigens are molecules the body identifies as non-self. They frequently are infecting organisms. However, they also can be part of a normal or cancerous cell in the body itself.

Antibodies are substances the body produces when it detects antigens inside it. They belong to a group of proteins called globulins. Since antibodies are involved in the body's immune system, they are referred to as immunoglobins (Ig).

TYPES OF IMMUNITY

Immunoglobins appear in your body in four ways. Some are acquired naturally while others are introduced to your body.

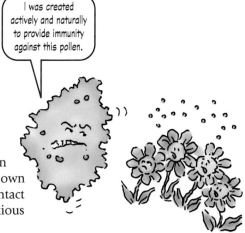

I was created actively and naturally to provide immunity against this pollen.

Active Natural Immunity

Active natural immunity occurs when people are exposed to a foreign antigen as a natural process and develop their own antibodies to fight it. Examples are contact with pollen in the air or with an infectious virus or bacteria.

Active Induced Immunity

Active induced immunity occurs when a person is exposed to a foreign antigen as part of therapy and develops his own antibodies to fight it. Examples are injections of mumps or measles vaccines.

Passive Natural Immunity

Passive natural immunity occurs when infants receive already-made antibodies from their mothers. These antibodies cross from mother to fetus in the placenta. They are also found in the milk of nursing mothers, especially in first two weeks after delivery.

Passive Induced Immunity

Passive induced immunity occurs when a person receives already-made antibodies as part of therapy. Examples are RhoGAM

(Rh Immune Globin), given to Rh-negative mothers who have Rh-positive babies, and some rabies injections.

TYPES OF ANTIBODIES

There are five general groups of immunoglobins.

Immunoglobin M

Immunoglobin M (IgM) antibodies are the largest in size. They are also the first to appear when the body detects an antigen. IgM antibodies are fairly crude in that they are less specific to particular antigens than the second antibody to appear in an immune response, IgG. IgM antibodies don't cross the placental barrier. Therefore, they neither help nor harm a fetus or newborn child.

Immunoglobin G

Immunoglobin G (IgG) antibodies develop after IgM formation. They last longer than IgM and reach higher protective levels. Booster injections increase levels of IgG, and they last longer and longer following each booster. IgG can cross the placental barrier, allowing a mother to pass her immunities to her fetus. This protection remains good for about six months after birth, while the child's own immune system is developing.

Immunoglobin E

Immunoglobin E (IgE) antibodies function mainly in reaction to intestinal worms (called helminths) and allergic antigens. IgE stimulates the body to release a protein that's toxic for helminths. They also stimulate the release of histamine and other chemicals in allergic reactions. IgE actions are also responsible for a severe allergic reaction called anaphylactic shock.

Immunoglobin A

Immunoglobin A (IgA) is found in many secretions, such as mucus, tears, saliva, and breast milk. These antibodies combat microbes in body secretions and give nursing babies some of the mother's immunities.

Immunoglobin D

Immunoglobin D (IgD) antibodies are found on the surface of some inactive lymphocytes. The small amount present in blood serum is thought to result from the death of the lymphocyte cells. The function of IgD is unknown.

Immunology Testing

Immunology testing involves looking for antigens or antibodies in different types of body fluids, such as blood, urine, spinal fluid, and other fluids. Here are some of the conditions immunology tests can identify:

- bacterial and viral infections, such as hepatitis A and B, strep, human immunodeficiency virus (HIV), rubella, and Epstein-Barr virus
- chlamydia, syphilis, and Rocky Mountain spotted fever
- pregnancy in women, drugs in urine specimens, and hormones in serum
- blood types for donors and recipients

Most immunology testing involves the part of the blood called serum. This is why immunology is also known as **serology.** When blood is centrifuged, it separates into three parts:

- serum or plasma, which is the most liquid part of blood. It contains mostly water and the antibodies.
- the buffy coat, which is the middle layer of centrifuged blood. It contains the white blood cells and platelets.
- red blood cells, which are also called erythrocytes. They are the heaviest part of the blood.

Immunohematology is the testing that blood banks do on red blood cells (RBCs) and serum or plasma. This is done to make sure that blood from a **donor** (a person who contributes blood) matches the blood of the person who receives it. Many other immunology tests are performed in the POL.

ANTIGENS AND ANTIBODIES

Antigens can enter the body from the outside or they can occur within the body itself. Here are some examples:

- foreign substances from the environment, such as pollen, bacteria, or viruses
- the hormone the body produces that is detected in a positive pregnancy test
- proteins in the membranes of the RBCs that cause differences in people's blood (called "blood types")

When the body detects antigens, it produces antibodies. The antibodies then float through the bloodstream and bind with antigens they encounter. This binding is the first part of the body's process for destroying the antigens.

Each antibody is designed to recognize and bind with only one kind of antigen. This is called **specificity.** That antigen may be common to a related group of substances, or it may be unique to a specific substance. The smaller the group of substances in which the antigen can be found, the more specific the antibody is for it.

Antibodies are named after the specific antigen they're attracted to and by adding the prefix *anti-*. For example, if one type of antigen is called *A*, the antibodies attracted to it are known as *anti-A*.

Antibodies have a strong attraction to their antigens. Therefore, only a little of the antigen needs to be in a patient's lab sample for the antibody to find it. This is called **sensitivity.** Test manufacturers try to increase sensitivity through their tests' content and procedures. For example, temperature and the strength of a solution can affect sensitivity. That's why it's important to follow test procedures closely. Failure to do this can cause false results.

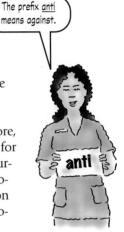

The prefix <u>anti</u> means against.

anti

IMMUNOLOGY TEST METHODS

Immunology testing is based on this attraction of specific antibodies to specific antigens. Here's how it works.

- You can test for the presence of specific antibodies in the patient by mixing a known antigen with the patient's sample and seeing if there's a reaction. This method is used to test patients for infectious mononucleosis, rheumatoid arthritis, syphilis, and rubella.

- You can test for the presence of a certain antigen in a patient by mixing its antibody with the patient's sample and seeing if there's a reaction. This method is used in some tests for strep infections, such as strep throat.

Most immunology tests are sensitive enough to detect fairly small amounts of antigens or antibodies in a patient's sample that contains millions of other substances. In some cases, the amount of the antigen or antibody present in the patient's sample is measured too.

The reagents used to conduct these tests contain antigens or antibodies that are specific to the kind of test being run. They also contain other substances that allow the test results to be observed. Because the binding of antigens and antibodies usually can't be seen by the naked eye, the reagents also provide ways to make the results more visible. They do this in two main ways.

- Agglutination tests depend on clumping to create visible particles if binding of antigens and antibodies occurs.

- Enzyme-linked immunosorbent assays (ELISA) rely on color changes to show positive or negative results.

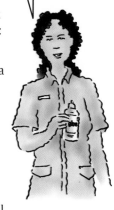

Think of the word glue to help you remember that the term <u>agglutination</u> means clumping together.

Agglutination Tests

Agglutination means the clumping together of materials that are suspended in a liquid. Agglutination tests are fast and easy to do. They're also inexpensive. Here's all you need:

- the specimen to be tested
- a reagent containing a known antibody or antigen and a clumping agent such as latex beads

The reagent and the patient's blood, urine, or other specimen are mixed and observed to see if binding will take place.

- If agglutination doesn't occur, the solution will appear smooth and milky. In most cases, this is a negative finding—the substance being tested for isn't present in the specimen.
- If agglutination does occur, antigens and antibodies will bind on the latex beads. The solution will appear rough and grainy, with areas of clumped particles. This result shows that the patient's specimen contains the substance for which it's being tested.

Sometimes, the binding and clumping involves red blood cells (RBCs) instead of latex beads. You'll read about that kind of testing when blood typing is covered later in this chapter.

Because agglutination tests are so sensitive and specific, their results are very accurate. This means you're less likely to get false-positives or false-negatives when using these tests.

Some tests require the clumping to happen within a certain time period for the results to be positive.

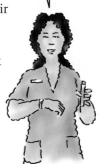

- A **false-positive** is a result that says a substance is present in a specimen when it actually is not.
- A **false-negative** is a result that fails to detect the substance being tested for, even though it's present in the specimen.

FALSE RESULTS

False results can have many causes. Some are biological conditions in the patient. Others are technical difficulties with samples or with performing the test. For example, here are some problems that can cause false-positive or false-negative results:

- waiting too long to look for agglutination or looking for it too soon
- **lipemic** samples (samples that have high fat levels)
- samples that have damaged RBCs, or hemolysis. Hemolysis is the rupture of red blood cell membranes. This results in the release of the constance of the red cell into the serum/plasma. Depending on the amount of hemolysis and tests ordered, a hemolyzed specimen may not be acceptable for testing.

You can't do much about the patient's biological condition, but you can avoid many technical problems by following directions carefully.

Enzyme-Linked Immunosorbent Assays

ELISA stands for enzyme-linked immunosorbent assays. (An assay is a test that analyzes the contents of a substance.) ELISA tests have more steps and more reagents than agglutination tests, but they result in an easy-to-read color change.

Most ELISA tests come in kits that contain all the reagents and other materials needed to run them. Some ELISA tests are so simple that all you have to do is put the patient's sample into

Closer Look   TEST RESULTS AND RETESTS

A false-positive on a lab test may show that a patient has a condition he really doesn't have. On the other hand, a false-negative might mean that a patient who actually has a problem will not get treatment for it.

False results can have serious effects for patients. False-positives could lead to treatments a patient doesn't need, which might even harm him. False-negatives can harm patients by delaying needed treatments.

When a test's results are positive, a patient's physician may order a second test before beginning treatment. This could be a different type of test or a repeat of the first test. Its purpose is to double-check the accuracy of the first test's results. If a patient's symptoms cast doubt on the accuracy of a negative result, the physician may order further testing in that case too.

a cartridge provided in the kit. The color changes if the sample contains the substance for which you're testing.

An assay can analyze a substance's contents, determine a drug's potency, and find out how much of something is present in a specimen.

Handling Test Reagents

Most immunology tests come in kits from a test manufacturer. These kits contain the reagents needed for the test. Many kits also include the pipettes, tubes, cups, and other things needed for the test to be done.

STORING REAGENTS

Reagent kits must be stored at the temperature the manufacturer states on the kit box or package insert. Some kits can be stored at room temperature (68 to 72 degrees F or 20 to 22 degrees C). Others will have to be kept in the lab refrigerator at 40 to 45 degrees F (4 to 8 degrees C). Some kits will have to be divided, with some reagents kept at room temperature and others in the refrigerator.

Be sure to read the instructions that come with each kit, so you'll know how to store its contents. If reagents are not stored properly, their quality may be affected. Poor-quality reagents may produce false results if you use them in testing.

If there's a problem with a test kit, its lot number can help you trace the trouble with the manufacturer.

GOOD PRACTICES WITH REAGENTS

Each reagent kit is marked with a lot number and expiration date. Kits with the same lot number were manufactured in the same place and at the same time. Only use reagents from kits that have the same lot number. Reagents from kits with different lot numbers shouldn't be used together. Manufacturers won't guarantee a test will work correctly if reagents from different lots are used.

PROPER USE OF REAGENTS

Here are some other tips for using reagents properly.

- Always check the expiration date on the kit box before using any of its reagents. Never use a reagent past its expiration date.

- When you open a new test kit, write the date and your initials on it. Some kits have a new expiration date that starts from the day they're opened.
- Always read the kit's package insert for details about handling its reagents and supplies.
- There may be guidelines with the kit for collecting or handling patient specimens. Be sure to read and follow these instructions.
- Check to make sure the manufacturer or supplier shipped the kits or reagents as recommended. For example, when requesting a delivery, make sure the package doesn't arrive on an afternoon when the office may be closed.

QUALITY CONTROL

Reagents don't always function correctly, even if they haven't expired. Here are a couple of ways this might happen.

- The reagent is properly stored in the refrigerator when you go to use it. However, a past user left it out too long and it got to room temperature before he put it back.
- A past user accidentally added serum or another solution to the reagent. This changed its composition so that it won't act correctly.

Quality Control for Test Kits

Kits should be tested regularly to make sure their reagents are performing correctly. Here are some basic guidelines for a good quality control (QC) program for test kits.

- A QC test should be done each time a kit's reagents are used.
- Some forms of QC may be needed when a new kit is opened.
- Other forms of QC may be performed daily.

Your lab also should have its own QC policies and procedures to follow. They will tell you exactly what the standards are for each step of each process.

External Controls

An **external control** is a solution that is used instead of a patient's sample during a QC test. The contents of the control

Closer Look — FOLLOWING TEST PROCEDURES

All immunology tests should have written procedures. To ensure correct results, you should follow them each time you test a sample. Test procedures usually cover these points:

- the test's clinical use
- the principles on which the test is based
- precautions to take in performing the test
- collecting and handling test specimens
- controls to be run and how often to run them
- step-by-step procedures
- interpreting and reporting results
- normal or expected values
- the test's limitations

solution are known, so if the reagent is okay, the test results should be as expected. Since the contents of the control solution are always the same, the test results should always be the same too. External controls are often part of test kits. In some cases, additional controls can be bought from the test manufacturer.

Checking most immunology test kits requires using negative controls as well as positive controls.

- When the test kit is run with the positive control, there should be a positive reaction. For example, if it's an agglutination test, clumping should occur. The correct color should appear if an ELISA is being tested.
- When the negative control is used, there should be no reaction—no agglutination or no color.

If external controls don't give the expected results, the results of any patient samples tested with the kit shouldn't be reported. This is because those results may not be accurate. Instead, the QC test should be repeated. If it again fails to perform correctly, the problem should be investigated.

Internal Controls

Some tests have **internal controls** that are built into the tests themselves. Each of these tests has test zones or areas that are separate from the zone or area for the specimen being

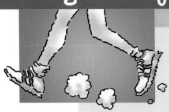

Running Smoothly

TROUBLESHOOTING TESTING PROBLEMS

What if a QC test doesn't do what it should?

You ran a QC test on a test kit and the test failed to perform correctly. You repeated the test and it produced incorrect results the second time too. Here are some steps to take to solve the problem.

1. First, check the reagents for signs of poor quality, like cloudiness or a change in color.

2. Next, reread the test procedure to make sure no steps were left out.

3. Then, check the labels on the reagents to make sure the right ones were added and in the correct order.

4. If none of these steps reveal the problem, repeat the test using a new control.

5. If the results are still incorrect, repeat the test again with a new test kit.

6. If the problem still exists, call the test manufacturer for advice.

7. After all problems have been resolved, report your results.

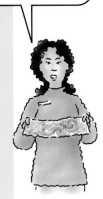

If the results are not correct even after you followed the correct steps, repeat the test.

tested. Some tests have a positive test zone and a negative test zone. Other tests have only a positive zone or a test-completed zone.

- The positive zone is a control to make sure the correct reagents were used in the test and in the proper order.

- The negative zone is a control to show if any abnormal reactions took place between the specimen and the reagents. That could mean a reagent was defective.

Each control zone must be checked for the proper reaction before the patient's test results are reported.

- The positive zone must give a positive color reaction.

- The proper reaction for the negative zone is no reaction at all. This usually means that no color appears.

The proper results in each control zone ensure that the correct procedure was followed when the patient specimen was tested and that the reagents worked properly.

So Many Tests!

There are many immunology tests. The next few pages will describe some of the ones most commonly done in a POL. These include tests for:

- rheumatoid arthritis
- infectious mononucleosis
- syphilis
- pregnancy
- strep infections

TESTING FOR RHEUMATOID ARTHRITIS

Rheumatoid arthritis (RA) is an **autoimmune disease** that affects the joints. (An autoimmune disease is a disease caused by a person producing antibodies against their own cells or tissue.) It progresses over time and inflames the joints, causing a lot of pain, stiffness, and swelling. RA has been linked to antibodies called rheumatoid factors. Testing a person's blood for these antibodies helps in diagnosing the disease.

The most common tests for rheumatoid factor are based on agglutination of particles. For test results to be valid, the positive control must agglutinate and the negative control must not agglutinate. If this is what happens, the results can be reported to the patient's physician.

Even when the controls act properly, lab tests are not perfect tools for diagnosing RA. Only about 70 percent of RA patients test positive for rheumatoid factor. The other 30 percent have a false-negative result. For this reason, physicians also use physical findings to make clinical decisions about the disease.

Test results also can be positive when the patient doesn't have RA. This is most likely to happen if the patient is elderly or has lupus, syphilis, or certain kinds of hepatitis.

TESTING FOR THE "KISSING DISEASE"

Infectious mononucleosis is commonly known as "mono" and even the "kissing disease." It's caused by the Epstein-Barr virus. The symptoms are fatigue, swollen lymph glands, sore throat, and sometimes other symptoms. It's fairly infectious and can be transmitted through saliva and other body fluids. Mono is sometimes called the kissing disease because that's one way it can spread.

The most common tests for mono include:

- agglutination of RBCs (Heterophile)
- agglutination of latex particles
- ELISA

SYPHILIS TESTS

The basic test for syphilis is called a rapid plasma reagin or RPR. RPR is an agglutination test. The patient's blood sample is tested for antibodies and antibody-like substances called reagins. If the test result is positive, the serum sample is diluted repeatedly, starting with a 1:2 ratio, then a 1:4, 1:8, 1:16 and so on.

The reason for this process is to find the weakest **titer** that will produce a positive reaction. A titer is the concentration or amount of a substance in a solution. For example, if the weakest dilution that shows agglutination is 1:8, the titer is listed as 1:8 when the results are reported.

The RPR is only a screening test. If its results are positive, tests that are more specific are done. These tests look for *Treponema pallidum*, the organism that causes syphilis, in the patient's blood. The two tests used to confirm a positive RPR are:

- MHA-TP, which stands for microhemagglutination assay for *T. pallidum*
- FTA-ABS, which stands for fluorescent treponemal antibody absorption test

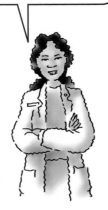

Patients with rheumatoid arthritis, lupus, mono, and hepatitis can falsely test positive for syphilis on an RPR. So can women who are pregnant.

These two tests are not performed in a POL. The patient's serum is sent to a reference lab (or to a state health department lab) for this testing.

There are four stages of syphilis. Only during the first two stages is the disease highly infectious.

- An RPR can detect antibodies in 80 percent of patients with first-stage syphilis. The other 20 percent will have false-negative results.
- An RPR is 99 percent effective in detecting second-stage syphilis. Only one percent of patients with the disease will have a false-negative test result at this stage.

Poor lab technique—improper rotation of the specimen during the test—can cause a false-negative result.

Legal Brief

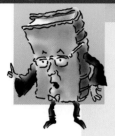

RAPID PLASMA REAGIN REPORTING REQUIREMENTS

A positive RPR for syphilis must be reported to the local health department. Public health authorities will contact the patient for his or her sexual history. The patient's sexual partners will then be warned so they can be tested.

If syphilis is undetected and untreated, it can cause major health problems and even death. These factors and the way it's spread would make it a serious public health problem if reporting requirements didn't exist.

PREGNANCY TESTS

Fertile women are often tested to rule out pregnancy before starting a medical procedure that could harm a fetus. Pregnancy tests are based on detecting the hormone HCG (human chorionic gonadotropin). Today's tests are so sensitive that they can determine pregnancy before a woman misses her first period. The tests for HCG include agglutination and ELISA. The Hands

Ask the Professional

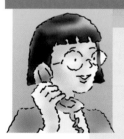

DEALING WITH AN AWKWARD SITUATION

Q: *One of our lupus patients was told that she has syphilis. Understandably, she was very upset. Now it turns out that she doesn't have it after all. How do we explain this mistake?*

A: First of all, you should be sensitive to how upsetting the test report must have been to her. Gently explain that mistakes can happen, even with the most accurate of tests. Although it may not be easy, you should try to give her the following information:

Explain that false positives can sometimes show up with diseases like lupus. When she came in for an STD test and it was positive, that was no real proof to assume she did not have it. You might tell her that even pregnant women and the elderly can show false positives on this test. The only way to know for sure is by further testing when there is any question about a diagnosis.

On feature on page 132 provides a step-by-step procedure for performing a pregnancy test in the lab.

A woman's first urine in the morning is the best urine specimen for the test. It's the most likely to contain HCG if she's pregnant. Urine that's too dilute can give a false-negative result. A false-positive for pregnancy can result if the woman has fibroids. That's because certain fibroid tumors produce HCG.

Testicular tumors produce HCG too and also give a false-positive result. So don't be surprised if you're asked to do a pregnancy test on a male patient. The physician may be trying to rule out a testicular tumor.

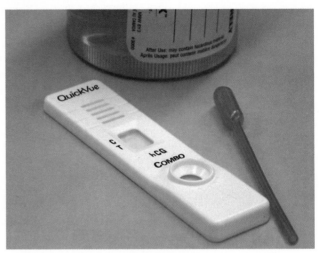

The QuickVue is one of many pregnancy assays that test urine specimens.

STREP TESTS

Group A streptococcus is one of the most common bacterial causes of sore throat and upper respiratory infections. Two types of tests are used for diagnosing strep infections. One is a serology test. The other is a culture. In both, you obtain the specimen by swabbing the patient's throat.

When you're getting a specimen from a patient who might have strep, collect two swabs in case the physician wants to do a culture.

The serology test is a rapid strep test. It can detect the bacteria even if they're not alive. One advantage of this test is that it can be done in 5 to 15 minutes. This allows the physician to begin treatment immediately if results are positive.

Culturing the specimen to see if bacteria grow from it takes 18 to 24 hours. However, a culture is the more sensitive and accurate test. If a rapid strep test is negative, the physician may send another specimen to the lab for a culture.

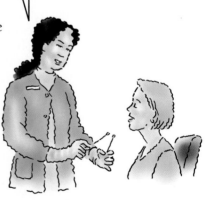

If you don't use proper technique to obtain the throat swab, the test results could be affected. Other reasons for false results in rapid strep tests and cultures are:

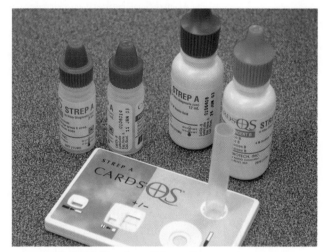

- not obtaining enough specimen
- swabbing the wrong area
- a high level of staph in the specimen
- letting the test stand too long before reading the results

Cards QS Strep A test kit is a rapid strep serology test.

Refer to the Hands On procedure on page 133 for instructions on how to perform a rapid strep test.

Blood Typing

You may remember from reading Chapter 1 that a lab's immunohematology department is also known as the blood bank. Blood to be transfused into a patient must be tested first to make sure it's compatible with the patient's blood. If it's not, the patient's body will treat it as a foreign substance and begin destroying it. This could lead to the patient's death!

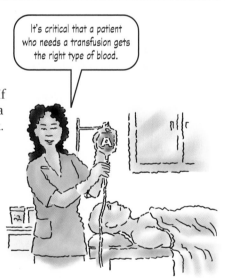

It's critical that a patient who needs a transfusion gets the right type of blood.

BLOOD GROUP ANTIGENS

Red blood cells (RBCs) contain antigens. The kind of antigens on a person's RBCs determines that person's blood type.

Every person belongs to one of four blood groups: A, B, O, or AB. Their blood group depends on what antigens are on their blood's RBCs. Here's how the blood groups are divided in the United States.

- About 40 percent of people have A blood.
- Some 11 percent of people are B.

- Some 45 percent of people have O blood.
- About four percent of people are AB.

The ABO Group

Almost everyone has antibodies to the RBC antigens that he or she lacks. These antibodies occur naturally in the body. Here's how it works:

- A person in the A blood group will have the A antigen *and* antibodies to type B blood.
- A person in the B blood group will have the B antigen *and* antibodies to type A blood.
- The AB person has *both* A and B antigens and does *not* have antibodies to either type A or type B.
- A person with O blood has *neither* the A nor B antigens, but antibodies to *both* types A and B.

Having antibodies to other types of blood prevents a patient from getting a transfusion using those types of blood. The antibodies in the patient's blood will cause her body to treat the new blood as a foreign substance and reject it. If the patient is transfused with blood to which she has no antibodies, her body will accept it. The table below summarizes this information for you.

Blood Group Donors and Recipients

Blood Group	Antigens	Antibodies	Can Receive Blood from	Can Give Blood to
A	A	Anti-B	A, O	A, AB
B	B	Anti-A	B, O	B, AB
AB	A and B	None	A, B, O	AB
O	None	Anti-A, Anti-B	O	A, B, AB, O

As you can see from the table, people with AB blood can have blood from any group transfused into them. The reason is that their blood has no A or B antibodies. However, they can give blood to only AB recipients. All the other blood groups have antibodies to their antigens.

On the other hand, people with O blood can receive blood only from O donors. That's because their blood contains antibodies to all the other blood groups. However, O blood can be given to patients of all blood types. For this reason, it is known as the universal donor.

Even though O blood has no antigens, some people with other blood types can still react badly to it. To prevent this, plasma is removed from the donor O blood and only the cells are transfused.

The Rh Group

A group of antigens called Rh is also important to the blood bank. Within the Rh group are several antigens. Of these antigens, D is the most important. Not all people have this antigen, however. The presence or absence of the D antigen in a person's blood determines what's called the **Rh factor.**

- When the D antigen is present, the blood is called Rh positive.
- When the D antigen is *not* present, the blood is called Rh negative.

Antibodies to D don't occur naturally. A person without the D antigen must be exposed to blood that has D for anti-D antibodies to develop in his body. This would happen if a patient with Rh-negative blood (blood without D) was transfused with Rh-positive blood (blood that contains the D antigen). The patient's body would form antibodies against the "foreign" D antigen and try to destroy the RBCs in the new blood.

So you can see that a person's Rh factor is another thing besides his ABO group to consider when doing transfusions. In some cases, mixing blood with different Rh factors can be life threatening, even when the ABO group of the blood is the same.

The best example of this is when a woman who is Rh negative becomes pregnant with an Rh-positive baby. (This can happen if the baby's father is Rh positive.) She will produce antibodies against the D antigens in the blood of her fetus. This can endanger the baby, especially if it's not her first Rh-positive child.

When an Rh-negative mother gives birth to an Rh-positive child, she is given a RhoGAM injection. RhoGAM must also be given within 72 hours to any Rh-negative woman whose pregnancy is terminated by miscarriage, still birth, or abortion. The RhoGAM prevents the mother from producing antibodies that might endanger her next baby by destroying its RBCs.

Other Blood Antigens

The ABO and Rh groups are the most important groups to immunohematology. There are other important blood antigens,

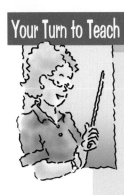

EXPECTANT MOTHERS AND RHOGAM

If you work with pregnant women who are Rh negative, you may need to inform them about RhoGAM injections. Here are some suggestions.

- First, explain to the patient's level of understanding what it means to be Rh negative.
- Explain that if the father is Rh positive or has an unknown Rh factor, the baby could have Rh-positive blood. (Also note that if the father has Rh-negative blood, there shouldn't be any need for RhoGAM.)
- Explain that if the baby's blood comes in contact with her blood, she'll make antibodies against the baby's blood. In future pregnancies, these antibodies will work against the fetal blood if it is Rh positive. This can cause severe hemolytic anemia, which can be fatal to the baby.
- Inform the patient that RhoGAM is a treatment to prevent her from producing these antibodies. It's given during and after labor. Tell her that she'll need to sign a consent form to have this treatment.
- Tell the patient that if she miscarries or has an abortion, she will still need RhoGAM.

Be aware that some doctors will automatically give *all* Rh-negative mothers RhoGAM. This avoids any awkward questions about who is the father of the child.

however. Here are some other groups of RBC antigens you may come across from time to time.

- Duffy
- Lewis
- MNS
- Kidd
- Kell

White blood cells (WBCs) and platelets also have antigens. Most of these are part of a system called human leukocyte antigens. A patient's antibodies to these antigens can cause fever during a blood transfusion. Antibodies to these antigens are also responsible when a patient rejects a transplanted organ, such as a heart or kidney.

BLOOD TYPE TESTING

Two lab tests are used to determine the ABO group of patients and of donor blood. A separate test can determine the blood's Rh. All three tests are agglutination tests. Their results reveal the blood type of a patient or donor blood.

Direct Typing

The direct way of finding out someone's ABO group is by using reagent antisera. This is serum that contains anti-A or anti-B antibodies. To do the test, the specimen's RBCs are diluted with **saline** (a solution of salt and water). Then a drop of the saline-RBC solution is mixed with a drop of anti-A antisera in a glass tube labeled A. Another drop is mixed with anti-B antisera in a tube labeled B. Both tubes are centrifuged for 15 seconds at a slow speed. The RBC sediment on the bottom of each tube is gently mixed again and examined for agglutination.

The illustration to the right shows the possible outcomes of this test and what each one means. Here they are in list form as well.

- If the RBCs in the A tube agglutinate, but not in the B tube, the blood is in the A group.

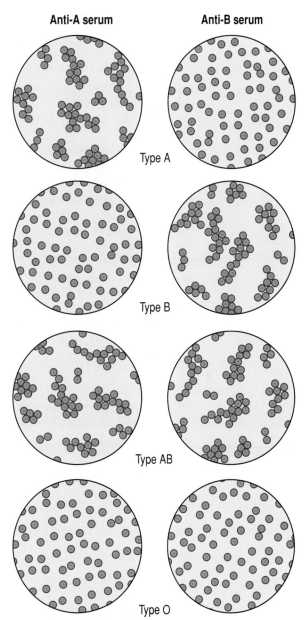

Anti-A serum   **Anti-B serum**

Type A

Type B

Type AB

Type O

Direct typing of blood: RBCs in type A blood are agglutinated only by anti-A serum. Those in type B blood are agglutinated only by anti-B serum. Type AB blood is agglutinated by both anti-A and anti-B. Type O is not agglutinated by either anti-A or anti-B.

- If the RBCs in the B tube agglutinate, but not in the A tube, the blood is in the B group.
- If the RBCs in both tubes agglutinate, the blood belongs to the AB group. This is because AB blood has both A and B antigens.
- If the RBCs don't agglutinate in either tube, the blood is in the O group. This is because O blood has no antigens.

Some labs call this method of typing blood forward typing instead of direct typing.

Indirect Typing

Indirect typing uses blood serum or plasma as the specimen instead of RBCs. (Remember that the serum in blood contains no red cells.) Reagents containing A-group cells and B-group cells are mixed with the specimen. The mix is centrifuged and examined for agglutination.

If the blood is A, for example, the serum specimen will contain only anti-B antibodies. Therefore, only the reagent with the B cells will agglutinate. If both reagents agglutinate, this means the serum specimen is from O blood. That's because O serum will contain both anti-A and anti-B antibodies.

This kind of testing is also called reverse typing. The table below summarizes the results for each blood group for both direct and indirect typing. A "positive" result means agglutination, while a "negative" result means no agglutination.

ABO Group Testing Results

Blood Group	Direct Typing Reagents		Indirect Typing Reagents	
	Anti-A	**Anti-B**	**A Cells**	**B Cells**
A	positive	negative	negative	positive
B	negative	positive	positive	negative
AB	positive	positive	negative	negative
O	negative	negative	positive	positive

Rh Testing

When testing for Rh factor, an anti-D reagent is used. The procedure is similar to the direct test for ABO typing.

- A drop of anti-D reagent is added to a drop of RBCs and saline in a test tube labeled D.

- The tube is centrifuged for 15 seconds.
- The RBCs are suspended again and observed for agglutination.
- If agglutination occurs, the blood is Rh positive. If not, it's Rh negative.

THE BLOOD SUPPLY

Blood banks often have a difficult time getting enough usable blood and blood products to meet the needs of recipients. There's a continuing shortage of volunteer donors. The American Red Cross and other agencies use bloodmobiles or worksites to collect blood.

Donating blood makes you feel good and helps others. Contact the American Red Cross for more information.

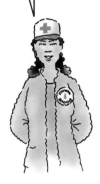

One 450-mL unit of donated whole blood can be divided into three products.

- Packed RBCs can be kept for 42 days if they're stored at a very low temperature. They are used to treat anemia.
- Plasma can be frozen and kept for up to a year. It's used to treat uncontrolled bleeding caused by lack of coagulation factors.
- Platelet concentrates are good for up to five days. They are stored at room temperature and are used to treat uncontrolled bleeding caused by damaged platelets or low platelet counts.

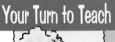

Your Turn to Teach

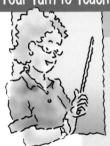

INSTRUCTING PERSONS WHO WANT TO DONATE BLOOD

The American Red Cross has rules for donating blood. These rules are based on government and other research. Each state also has laws that govern blood donations. You should check the laws in your own state.

Tell potential donors that, in general, they must meet following conditions:

1. at least 17 years old
2. weigh at least 110 lbs
3. have a hemoglobin level of at least 12.5 g/dL
4. have a pulse rate of 50 to 110 beats per minute

(continued)

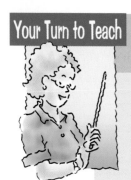

Your Turn to Teach

INSTRUCTING PERSONS WHO WANT TO DONATE BLOOD (*continued*)

5. have a blood pressure lower than 180 over 100

6. be willing and able to provide a brief medical history

The potential donor may ask you how long it will take to give blood. The actual donation time is only about 10 to 20 minutes. However, the entire process takes about an hour.

Blood can be donated every two months, and only one pint may be donated at a time. All donated blood is tested by the American Red Cross for HIV, hepatitis, syphilis, and at least 20 other conditions.

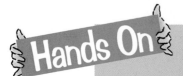

Hands On

PERFORMING AN HCG PREGNANCY TEST

4-1

Follow these steps to perform an assay on a patient's specimen for pregnancy. (Be aware that manufacturers' kits, timing, drops, and control procedures can vary from lab to lab. Follow office policies to ensure accuracy and quality control.)

1. Wash your hands.

2. Assemble the test kit's equipment. The kit should be at room temperature.

3. Check that the names on the specimen container and lab form are the same.

4. Use one test pack for the patient and one for each control.

5. Label the three test packs as follows: the patient's name, "positive control," and "negative control."

6. In the patient's chart and the control log, record the type of specimen you're obtaining (urine or plasma/serum).

7. Use a transfer pipette to aspirate the specimen. Place four drops in the sample well of the test pack labeled with the patient's name.

8. Carefully aspirate the positive control and place four drops in the sample well of the pack labeled "positive control."

9. Follow the exact same step for the negative control.

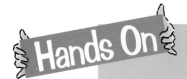

PERFORMING AN HCG PREGNANCY TEST (continued)

4-1

10. Consult the test manufacturer's insert in the kit to interpret test results. The insert will tell you what to look for in reading a positive or negative result.

11. Report the results when the end-of-assay window is read and after you have checked the controls for accuracy. This will happen at about seven minutes for serum and about four minutes for urine. The end-of-assay window should either change or appear wet. If it doesn't and/or the controls don't work, the test must be redone.

12. Record the controls and patient's information on the worksheet or log form and in the patient's records.

13. Clean up the work area and dispose of all waste properly.

Charting Example:
01/14/2007   16:00   Pt. complains of late period—
LMP 11/22/06. Complains of nausea in a.m., breast tenderness. Urine sample positive for pregnancy. Dr. Khoury examined pt. Pregnancy brochures explained to pt. RTC. _____
_____ J. Giles, CMA

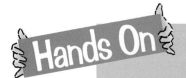

PERFORMING A GROUP A RAPID STREP TEST

4-2

Follow these steps to perform a Group A Rapid Strep Test. (Be aware that manufacturers' kits and control procedures can vary from lab to lab. Follow office policies to ensure accuracy and quality control.)

1. Wash your hands.

2. Double check that the names on the specimen container and the lab form are the same.

3. Label one extraction tube with the patient's name, one with "positive control," and one with "negative control."

4. Follow the kit directions. Carefully add the correct reagents and drops to each of the extraction tubes.

(continued)

Hands On

PERFORMING A GROUP A RAPID STREP TEST (*continued*)

4-2

5. Insert the patient's culture swab (which is one of the two swabs) into the labeled extraction tube. If only one swab was taken, first swab a beta strep agar plate. Then, use the same swab for the actual test.

6. Add the right controls to each of the two control tubes and place a sterile swab into each control tube.

7. Use the swab to mix each tube's contents by twirling each swab five to six times.

8. Set a timer for the amount of time specified by the manufacturer of the test.

9. Draw the swab up from the bottom of each tube and out of any liquid. Press out all fluid on the swab head by rolling the swab against the inside of the tube before it is withdrawn.

10. Add three drops from the well-mixed extraction tube to the sample window of the strep A test unit labeled with the patient's name. Do the same for each control.

11. Set the timer for the correct amount of time.

12. A positive result will show up as a line in the result window within five minutes.

13. A negative result is indicated if no line appears within five minutes. However, you must wait exactly five minutes to read a negative result, to avoid getting a false negative.

14. Verify the control results before recording any test results. Log the controls and the patient's information into your log or worksheet.

15. You may have to culture all negative rapid strep tests on a blood agar, if your lab requires it. (A bacitracin disk may be added to the first quadrant when you set up the blood agar.

16. Clean up the work area and dispose of all waste in the right place.

17. Don't forget to wash your hands!

Charting Example:
05/22/2007   11:15 A.M.   Pt. complains of sore throat × 2 days. Group A rapid strep test positive. Dr. Nguyen notified. _____
_____ A. Bailey, RMA

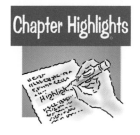

Chapter Highlights

- All serological testing includes how antigens and antibodies react.
- Specimens from patients can include many different kinds of body fluids, such as serum, urine, or spinal fluid.
- The most common types of tests are agglutination tests and ELISA.
- There are many types of test kits. You must be familiar with the steps involved in each one used in your lab.
- Each day that tests are performed, quality control (QC) processes must be strictly followed.
- You may have to arrange for your physician's patients to undergo transfusions at places outside the medical office. You must have a good understanding of ABO blood groups and Rh types to correctly answer any questions patients may have.

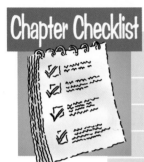

Chapter 5

URINALYSIS

Chapter Checklist

- Explain why urinalysis is done and summarize the medical assistant's involvement in this process
- Describe the methods of urine collection
- Obtain a clean-catch midstream urine specimen
- Explain how and why urine specimens are tested
- Perform a chemical reagent test strip analysis
- Explain what a urine culture is and why it is done
- Identify the physical properties of urine and note some conditions that can affect them
- Determine the color and clarity of urine
- List the main chemical substances that may be found in urine and explain what the presence of each might mean
- Perform a Clinitest
- Perform a nitroprusside reaction (ACETEST) for ketones
- Perform an acid precipitation test for proteins
- Perform the diazo tablet test (Icotest) for bilirubin
- Identify substances that might be found in urine sediment and describe how urine sediment is examined
- Prepare urine sediment
- Describe how urine pregnancy tests are conducted
- Describe how urine drug tests are conducted

Urinalysis involves examining and testing urine. Urine tests are often done in the physician office lab (POL). Many are CLIA-waived, meaning that medical assistants can perform them. Conducting these tests may be part of your duties as a medical assistant.

Another part of your job may be preparing urine specimens for other tests by the physician or other trained personnel. Knowing the basics of urinalysis will help you carry out these responsibilities.

Urinalysis and You

Urinalysis is part of the process the physician uses to assess a patient's health. Like blood testing, urinalysis can show things of which even the patient may not be aware.

Here are just some of the conditions that urine tests can reveal:

- liver disease
- kidney disease
- diabetes
- malnutrition
- dehydration
- infection
- pregnancy

SPECIMEN COLLECTION METHODS

Another part of your duties may be collecting specimens for testing. There are several ways to collect a urine specimen. The method used often depends on what test will be performed. Unless the physician tells you otherwise, a freshly voided specimen is usually all that's needed. This is called a random urine. The patient voids into a dry, clean container.

The time of collection is sometimes an important factor. The most concentrated urine is voided just after a person wakes up in the morning. Concentrated specimens are useful for many types of tests. For example, pregnancy tests are usually done with "first-morning" urine. Other timed tests are post-prandial, which means after a meal. Some post-prandial tests measure concentrations of glucose in urine collected two hours after the patient has eaten.

Clean Catch

Clean-catch midstream urine is the most commonly ordered random specimen. It is especially useful when an infection is suspected. That's because if the specimen is collected correctly, any microorganisms present will be from the urinary tract and not the result of contamination by the patient's skin or other factors.

A clean-catch urine specimen is sent to the laboratory in a clean, dry container with a lid. If the specimen is to be cultured, the container must also be sterile. A **culture** can then be performed to detect the microorganism that is causing the disease. A culture is a test in which bacteria and other microbes are grown in a lab. You'll read more about cultures later in this chapter and in Chapter 7.

Patients generally collect clean-catch specimens themselves. Since the correct collection procedure is so important to accurate test results, you'll often be instructing patients in the proper methods to use. Use the Hands On procedure on page 164 as a guide when doing this.

KEY POINTS ABOUT THE CLEAN-CATCH METHOD

Here are some of the key points to remember about the clean-catch collection method.

- Collection should be done after the urinary meatus and surrounding skin have been cleansed.
- The urine should be voided into a clean container. A sterile container must be used if a culture has been ordered.
- The specimen can be used as a culture only if nothing (such as a pipette or reagent strip) is allowed to contaminate the urine first.

Other Collection Methods

Both the type of test and the type of patient can affect how the specimen is collected. Most specimens are collected by a clean-catch midstream method. Other collection methods exist, but they are less common and generally require the direct involvement of a health care professional.

> As with other body fluids, you should wear proper protective gear and follow OSHA guidelines when handling urine specimens.

Bladder Catheterization. In *bladder catheterization,* a thin sterile tube called a catheter is inserted into the bladder through the urethra. Bladder catheterization is recommended when the patient can't give a urine specimen in a sterile manner using the clean-catch method.

Suprapubic Aspiration. Suprapubic aspiration is the least common method of urine collection. A needle is inserted into the bladder through the abdominal wall above the symphysis pubis, and urine is withdrawn. A physician performs this method in a surgical setting.

Collection Device. A collection device is usually used to collect urine from young children. You apply the device around the mons pubis or external genitalia and collect the urine in a bag.

COLLECTING URINE FROM INFANTS

When collecting a urine specimen from an infant or young child who isn't toilet-trained, you'll need to apply a collection device. The procedure should take five minutes.

Here's a list of the equipment you'll need.

- gloves
- personal antiseptic wipes
- pediatric urine collection bag
- completed laboratory request slip
- biohazard transport container

Follow these steps to correctly apply a urine collection device to an infant.

1. Gather the equipment and supplies and then wash your hands.
2. Explain the procedure to the parents.
3. Have the infant lie on her back. Ask for help from parents as needed.
4. After putting on gloves, clean the genitalia with the antiseptic wipes.
   A. For girls: Cleanse front to back with separate wipes for each downward stroke on the outer labia. The last clean wipe should be used between the inner labia.
   B. For boys: Retract the foreskin if the child isn't circumcised. Cleanse the meatus in an ever-widening circle. Discard the wipe and repeat the procedure. Return the foreskin to its proper position.
5. Holding the collection device, remove the upper portion of the paper backing and press it around the mons pubis. Remove the second section and press it against the perineum. Loosely attach a diaper.
6. Give the infant fluids unless it's otherwise indicated. Check the diaper frequently.

7. When the infant has voided, remove the collection device and diaper. Clean the skin of any adhesive that remains.

8. Prepare the specimen for transport to the laboratory or process it according to the office policy and procedure manual.

9. Remove your gloves and wash your hands.

10. Record the procedure in the patient's chart.

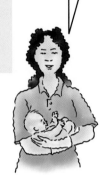

When collecting urine from an infant, enlist the parent's help. The infant will probably be more cooperative if a parent helps you with this procedure.

24-Hour Urine Collection. The amount of hormones and some other substances that are excreted in urine can vary during the day. Tests for these substances are more accurate when all urine is collected over a 24-hour period. You'll need to instruct patients about a 24-hour urine collection since it's usually done at home.

TESTING METHODS

Urinalysis includes both physical examination and chemical testing of urine. Before a specimen is tested, its appearance and odor are evaluated. Then the urine is tested for a number of things it might contain. Sometimes these tests lead to a third step in urinalysis—growing a culture of the specimen.

Physical Examination

Physical examination involves looking at the specimen to judge its color and how clear it is. Other observations include:

- measuring the specimen's specific gravity; this tells how concentrated the patient's urine is.

- looking at the specimen under a microscope; this provides information about

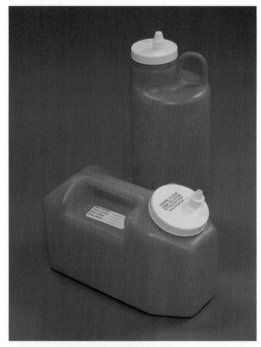

Here are two different styles of 24-hour urine collection containers that you might send home with a patient.

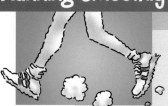

Running Smoothly — WHEN COLLECTING SPECIMENS FROM INFANTS

How can I protect myself from being accused of inappropriate behavior when applying a urine collection device?

Applying a urine collection device to an infant can involve some legal risks. To prevent possible accusations of fondling or other inappropriate behavior, always have a parent present during the procedure. In addition, be sure to explain clearly to the parent what you're going to do before you do it. It's also a good idea to have the parent assist with the process and help keep the infant calm.

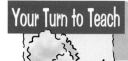

Your Turn to Teach — INSTRUCTING PATIENTS IN 24-HOUR URINE COLLECTION

Give the following instructions to patients who must perform a 24-hour urine collection.

General Instructions

- Follow these instructions exactly. Your test results are based on the total amount of urine excreted by your body over a 24-hour period. If you don't follow these instructions carefully, the test results may be inaccurate.
- Before you start the collection, check with the physician or lab for any dietary or drug restrictions.
- Make sure you drink the amount of fluid you normally would during the 24-hour collection period.
- Use the special container you are given to collect the urine. If a preservative is in the container, don't throw it away.
- Preservatives may be caustic or toxic. Be careful not to spill the preservative. If you do spill the preservative, immediately wash with large amounts of water. Then, call the physician or lab to get a new container to collect the specimen.

(continued)

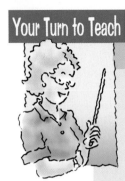

INSTRUCTING PATIENTS IN 24-HOUR URINE COLLECTION (*continued*)

- Don't void directly into the container unless a funnel is provided. Instead, use the collection cups you are given and transfer their contents to the large container. Collect your urine often enough that the amount you void each time doesn't exceed the volume of the collection cup.

- Refrigerate the container during collection. The urine must be kept cold.

Instructions for Day 1

- When you wake up in the morning, empty your bladder into the toilet. Record the date and the exact time (to the minute) on your 24-hour urine container.

- Then, collect all specimens during the day, evening, and night for the next entire 24-hour period.

- Add all the specimens to the container. Be careful not to get the cap of the container wet.

- Keep the container refrigerated until you take it to the physician or lab for testing.

Instructions for Day 2

- Exactly 24 hours after you began, completely empty your bladder and add this specimen to the container. This will be your last collection.

- Record the ending date and the exact time (to the minute) on the container.

- Replace the cap and tighten firmly.

- Refrigerate the specimen until you can turn it in. Take the specimen to the physician or lab as soon as possible.

- If you were under any dietary restrictions, you may resume your normal diet after you finish collecting your specimen.

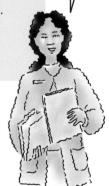

Remember to document any patient education and instructions given to the patient in the patient's chart.

cells, bacteria, and other tiny objects that may be in a patient's urine.

Chemical Testing

The basic urine test typically uses a strip with ten pads spread along its surface. A reagent in each pad tests for a

Closer Look   PRESERVING SPECIMENS FOR TESTING

Urine specimens generally should be tested within an hour after they're collected because the specimen will begin deteriorating after that time. The microorganisms in the urine will multiply, causing it to change from acidic to alkaline. The microorganisms also may consume glucose in the urine as a nutrient. This will lower the specimen's glucose level. A glucose test in this case would not be measuring the true level of glucose in the patient's urine.

If testing won't be performed within an hour, you should refrigerate the container at 4 to 8 degrees C (39 to 46 degrees F). This will slow down changes in the specimen. Urine may be refrigerated for up to four hours and still be good enough for accurate testing.

specific substance in urine. The pads change color when the strip is dipped in the specimen. The color each pad becomes reveals if that substance is present in the specimen.

Each pad's color is compared to a color chart provided by the strip's manufacturer. An example of one manufacturer's color chart is on page 144. Each row on the chart corresponds to one pad on the strip. You can see the ten things for which this manufacturer's reagent strip tests. You also can see that in most cases, the test result gives a rough estimate of how much of the substance is present in the specimen.

The Hands On procedure on page 166 provides step-by-step directions for testing urine with reagent strips. Instead of the manual reading of reagent strips, your facility may have an automated strip reader. In that case, follow the manufacturer's directions for machine operation. These tests are basic screening tests only. To confirm a result, or if more specific information is needed, higher level follow-up testing is done in many cases.

Urine Cultures

Chemical testing results and microscopic examination may suggest that a patient's urine contains large amounts of bacteria. This generally means that the patient has a urinary tract infection (UTI). Before the infection can be treated, the organism causing it must be identified. To do this, the urine specimen is cultured.

A small amount of the specimen is inoculated onto a plate that's been filled with **media**—a substance containing

2161

Multistix® 10 SG

Reagent Strips for Urinalysis
For In Vitro Diagnostic Use

READ PRODUCT INSERT BEFORE USE.
IMPORTANT: Do not expose to direct sunlight.
Do not use after 1/08.

COLOR CHART

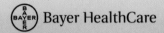

Bayer HealthCare

TESTS AND READING TIME

Test						
LEUKOCYTES 2 minutes	NEGATIVE	TRACE	SMALL +	MODERATE ++	LARGE +++	
NITRITE 60 seconds	NEGATIVE	POSITIVE	POSITIVE	(Any degree of uniform pink color is positive)		
UROBILINOGEN 60 seconds	NORMAL 0.2	NORMAL 1	mg/dL 2	4	8	(1 mg = approx. 1EU)
PROTEIN 60 seconds	NEGATIVE	TRACE	mg/dL 30 +	100 ++	300 +++	2000 or more ++++
pH 60 seconds	5.0	6.0	6.5	7.0	7.5	8.0	8.5
BLOOD 60 seconds	NEGATIVE	NON-HEMOLYZED TRACE	NON-HEMOLYZED MODERATE	HEMOLYZED TRACE	SMALL +	MODERATE ++	LARGE +++
SPECIFIC GRAVITY 45 seconds	1.000	1.005	1.010	1.015	1.020	1.025	1.030
KETONE 40 seconds	NEGATIVE	mg/dL	TRACE 5	SMALL 15	MODERATE 40	LARGE 80	LARGE 160
BILIRUBIN 30 seconds	NEGATIVE	SMALL +	MODERATE ++	LARGE +++		
GLUCOSE 30 seconds	NEGATIVE	g/dL (%) mg/dL	1/10 (tr.) 100	1/4 250	1/2 500	1 1000	2 or more 2000 or more

©2001, 2003 Bayer HealthCare LLC, Diagnostics Division, Tarrytown, NY 10591   01   Rev. 1/06   0350110

This chart shows the possible color reactions for each of the ten pads on a reagent strip that's used to test urine. Results are obtained by comparing each reagent pad's color to the chart's colors for the same test.

things bacteria need to grow. (You'll learn more about this method in Chapter 7.) Next, the dish is incubated, or warmed, to make the bacteria grow faster. If there are bacteria in the specimen, colonies of bacteria will soon be visible to the naked eye in the culture dish. The culture can then be tested to find the right antibiotic to fight the patient's infection.

A doctor will usually start a patient on an antibiotic to kill bacteria that are the most common cause of UTIs, even before the culture is done. Then, when the culture results are known, the doctor may need to change the antibiotic if a type of bacteria is found that isn't killed by the antibiotic the patient has been taking.

When culturing urine, it's important that the specimen not be contaminated. Contamination can happen when the patient does not follow proper collection procedure. For example, bacteria could get into a clean-catch urine specimen if it came in contact with the patient's skin. Another way the specimen can become contaminated is if it's used for another test. In either case, it would produce false results in a urine culture.

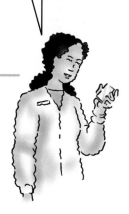

The media in urine cultures encourages the bacteria to grow rapidly until they can be seen with the naked eye.

Physical Properties of Urine

The physical properties of a patient's urine can tell you a lot about the patient's general health. Urine's physical properties include:

- color
- appearance (such as clear or cloudy)
- specific gravity
- odor

A specimen's odor may not be included in the urinalysis report. However, it can alert an experienced medical assistant to certain conditions. For example, a sweet odor can be a sign that the patient has diabetes. Bacteria in urine can make it smell foul or ammoniacal.

You'll determine the sample's color and clarity by visual inspection. Then you'll use your judgment to decide if they fall within the normal range. The Hands On procedure on page 168 tells how to check the color and clarity of a urine specimen. The normal range for urine's physical properties is shown in the table below.

Normal Range for Physical Properties of Urine

Property	Expected Range
Color	pale yellow to dark yellow
Clarity	clear
Odor	slightly aromatic
Specific gravity	1.003–1.035

COLOR

Urine's normal color ranges from pale straw color to dark yellow. Many things can affect its color, including:

- drugs
- diet

- disease

- its concentration

Pale colored urine usually means that it's diluted. This can happen if the patient has been drinking a lot of fluid. It also can result from diuretic therapy. **Diuretics** are drugs that increase the body's urine production. They're sometimes used to treat hypertension (high blood pressure). They're also prescribed to remove excess fluid from the body's tissues. This build up can result from kidney, lung, liver, or heart disease. The removed fluid dilutes the urine, making it paler in color.

Dark yellow urine can mean that it's highly concentrated. This can be a sign that the patient is dehydrated. It also can mean that the patient recently took a multivitamin pill. Foods such as blackberries, rhubarb, beets, and those with red dye can cause dark or reddish urine that might look like **hematuria,** or blood in the urine. The table below shows some other common causes of various colors of urine.

Common Causes of Color Variations in Urine

Color	Possible Causes
Yellow-brown or amber	bilirubin in urine (as in jaundice)
Dark yellow	concentrated urine, low fluid intake, dehydration, inability of kidney to dilute urine, fluorescein (intravenous dye), multivitamins, excessive carotene
Bright orange-red	Pyridium (urinary tract analgesic)
Red or reddish-brown	hemoglobin pigments, pyrvinium pamoate (Povan) medication for intestinal worms, sulfonamides (sulfa-based antibiotics)
Green or blue	artificial color in food or drugs
Blackish, grayish, smoky	hemoglobin or remains of old red blood cells (indicating bleeding in upper urinary tract), chyle, prostatic fluid, yeasts, homogentisic acid

CLARITY

Urine is normally clear when it's voided. Urine that's **turbid** (cloudy) probably contains **particulate matter,** or tiny solid particles.

Urine samples that have been sitting a long time can turn cloudy from the **precipitation** (settling out) of phosphates and urates that are in the solution. **Phosphates** are compounds made of phosphorous and oxygen. **Urates** are nitrogen compounds that result when the body burns protein. Urine that's turbid for this reason is considered normal.

Other causes of turbidity may be a sign of problems. Here are some substances that can make urine turbid:

- white blood cells (WBCs)
- red blood cells (RBCs)
- epithelial cells (skin and organ-lining cells)
- pus
- mucus
- fat droplets
- blood
- bacteria

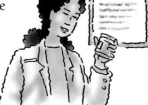

I'd say this specimen is looking pretty cloudy. What do you think?

Labs have their own ways for expressing how clear a urine specimen is. The most common terms are *clear, hazy,* and *cloudy*. A clear specimen container or a clear centrifuge tube containing the specimen is held up against a white paper with black lines on it.

- If the black lines can't be seen through the specimen, it's called *cloudy*.
- If the specimen is turbid but the lines can still be seen through it, the urine is judged to be *hazy*.

SPECIFIC GRAVITY

Specific gravity measures the concentration of urine. To find its specific gravity, the weight of urine is compared to the weight of water. Urine is normally slightly heavier than water. That's because it contains substances like sodium, potassium, and chloride, which water does not. This makes urine weigh more than the same amount of water would.

Specific gravity is not an actual weight, however. Instead, it's a comparison to the weight of water. The specific gravity of water is set at 1.000. Substances that are lighter than water (and which would float on it) have a specific gravity of less then 1.000—for example, 0.785. Things that are heavier than water have a specific gravity greater then 1.000. The specific gravity of a normal urine specimen will range between 1.003 and 1.035.

Urine that's dilute will have a lower specific gravity. As you've read, dilute urine can result if the patient has taken a lot of fluids. Abnormal conditions that cause dilute urine include diabetes insipidus and kidney infections.

Urine that has a high specific gravity is concentrated. A patient who's dehydrated could easily produce such a specimen. Dehydration can result from a number of conditions, including:

- heavy sweating
- prolonged vomiting
- frequent diarrhea

The body tries to conserve water when it becomes dehydrated. Therefore, the urine produced will be more concentrated.

Diabetes mellitus also can cause urine to have a high specific gravity. That's because of the high concentration of glucose the urine contains. IVP dye, the x-ray dye used to visualize the urinary system, can also cause urine to have a high specific gravity. This doesn't reflect the patient's state of hydration, but simply shows the presence of a foreign substance with a high weight. The specimen will frequently look clear and colorless, but have a high specific gravity.

Chemical Properties of Urine

Urine contains a number of chemicals. Some of these are produced by the body itself. Others are taken in from the

---

Closer Look   HOW URINE IS "WEIGHED"

Specific gravity is generally determined by one of three ways.

- *Reagent strip*—the specific gravity pad on a reagent test strip also takes just one drop of urine. The pad's change in color measures the urine's specific gravity. This is the most common method of determining specific gravity.
- *Urinometer*—this device looks something like an oral thermometer. It floats upright in the specimen and its upper part has a calibrated scale. The specific gravity is measured by how much of the device sinks into the urine.
- *Refractometer*—this device only requires a drop of urine, compared to about 100 mL that's needed to float a urinometer. It works by measuring how light passing through the urine drop is affected by the particles in it.

environment. The reagent strip test makes ten chemical measurements. The following table lists the expected or "normal" results for these tests. The chart on page 144 reveals what color each test pad should be to show the result listed in the table.

Expected Range of Urine's Chemical Properties

Property Tested for	Expected Range or Result
Glucose	negative
Bilirubin	negative
Ketones	negative
Blood	negative
pH	5.0–8.0
Protein	negative to trace
Urobilinogen	0.1–1.0 EU/dL
Nitrite	negative
Leukocyte esterase	negative

CONFIRMATION TESTS

A confirmation test is often ordered to follow up on a positive result on a strip test. These tests use a different chemical reaction to look for the substance than was used by the strip test. Confirmation tests are usually performed to make sure the results of the strip test are correct. Here are common confirmation tests for some chemicals found in urine:

- protein—sulfosalicylic acid test
- ketones—ACETEST
- bilirubin—Ictotest
- glucose—Clinitest

Some labs automatically do them when strip test results are abnormal. Your lab should have a written procedure on the performing of confirmation tests.

DETERMINING pH

The pH of urine is one of the things tested on the reagent strip. It is a measure of how acid or how alkaline (base) a liquid is. If a pH is greater than 7.0, the liquid is alkaline. Values less than 7.0 indicate acids. The higher or lower the number, the more alkaline or acidic the liquid is.

Acids are a product of the body's chemical processes. **Ammonia** is a base that's produced when nitrogen in the body breaks down. The kidneys clean the blood of these and other substances and get rid of them in urine. Urine is usually acidic because the body produces more acids than bases.

The pH of freshly voided urine is slightly acidic at 6.0. But the expected range for a normal pH is from 5.0 (acidic) to 8.0 (slightly alkaline). If the patient has a high-protein diet or uncontrolled diabetes, urine can be more acidic. Alkaline urine can occur after meals and in these situations:

- the patient follows a vegetarian diet
- the patient has certain renal (kidney) diseases
- the patient has a UTI

GLUCOSE TESTING

Glucose is filtered from the blood in the glomerulus of the kidney's nephron into the Bowman's capsule portion of the nephron. To conserve the glucose for the body, it is reabsorbed into the blood from the tubule portion of the nephron. However, the nephron can only reabsorb glucose up to a blood level of about 180 mg/dL. This is known as the *renal blood glucose threshold level.* If the blood glucose is higher than 180 mg/dL, the glucose in excess of 180 mg/dL will start to pass out of the nephron in the urine.

Normal urine does not contain glucose. It's rare that a healthy person's blood glucose level would exceed 180 mg/dL. **Glycosuria** (glucose in urine) can be a sign of diabetes or some other condition related to **hyperglycemia** (high blood sugar). Diabetics whose condition is uncontrolled or poorly managed may pass glucose in their urine because of a high level in their blood.

Clinitest

The copper reduction test method (Clinitest) can detect any reducing sugar in urine. Reducing sugars are sugars that give up electrons easily in chemical reactions. This type of sugars includes:

- glucose
- galactose
- lactose
- fructose

This test is often used to screen young children for **galactosuria,** or high levels of galactose in urine and blood. This condition results when a newborn lacks an enzyme that metabolizes

Closer Look   URINALYSIS AND DETECTING DIABETES

If a patient's blood glucose level is below 180 mg/dL, the urine reagent strip will test negative for glucose. Not until the blood level is above 180 mg/dL will the strip test show a positive result.

A fasting blood glucose level should be between 60 and 100 mg/dL. This is a fasting level, meaning that the person hasn't had anything to eat or drink for eight hours except water. Even after a meal, however, a healthy person's blood glucose level shouldn't reach the 180 mg/dL required for a positive urine strip test result.

Undetected or uncontrolled diabetes can lead to heart disease, kidney failure, blindness, and even death. Yet a person can be severely diabetic before signs will show up on a urine test. However, since a routine urinalysis is part of nearly every hospital admission and annual physical exam, it remains a primary method of screening for diabetes. The diagnosis is then confirmed by blood glucose tests.

Monitoring the glucose levels of known diabetics was also once done by urine testing. However, since the rise of handheld computerized glucose monitors in the 1980s, urine monitoring has been replaced by testing blood samples taken by finger stick.

galactose in the body. The Hands On procedure on page 169 gives you directions for performing a Clinitest.

Clinitest results can be inaccurate when used simply to confirm a positive strip test result for glucose. That's because other sugars and vitamin C in the specimen will also react with the

CLINITEST SAFETY

The Clinitest is a reagent test that produces a strong chemical reaction. This reaction gives off a large amount of heat. You should always use glass test tubes when performing this test. Never use plastic. Wait 15 seconds after the reaction stops before touching the tubes. This allows them time to cool. Finally, avoid touching the bottoms of the test tubes. They become very hot during the test.

reagent. However, a negative strip test result combined with a positive Clinitest result strongly suggests that the patient has a carbohydrate metabolism disorder.

> When performing a Clinitest, remember: those test tubes can get hot! Make sure the test tube is glass and not plastic. The plastic will melt.

TESTING FOR KETONES

Ketones are chemicals the body makes when it metabolizes fat. Most of your energy comes from carbohydrates. When the body doesn't have enough carbohydrates to meet its needs, it burns fats for energy. This happens if a person is starving or is eating a low-carbohydrate, high-protein diet. Poorly managed diabetics also get energy from fats and produce ketones.

Normally, there are too few ketones in urine to even measure. When a patient's urine tests positive for ketones, it's a sign his body is burning more fat than normal.

Nitroprusside is used to detect ketones in urine. Nitroprusside is a nitrogen-cyanic compound that reacts with ketones. It's used on reagent strips and in tablet tests. A tablet test called the ACETEST is used in many labs to confirm the results of the strip test. The Hands On procedure on page 172 tells you how to do an ACETEST.

TESTING FOR PROTEINS

A small amount of proteins is normal in urine. High amounts can be an important sign of renal disease. Other things that can cause protein in urine are:

- strenuous exercise
- pregnancy
- infection
- hematuria
- pyuria (white blood cells in the urine)
- multiple myeloma (a cancer of the bone marrow)
- orthostatic proteinuria

Examining urine under a microscope can help find whether high protein levels are caused by bacteria, casts, or cell-related factors. (You'll read about casts later in this chapter.)

Urine is screened for proteins on a reagent test strip. Results are confirmed with a turbidity or precipitation test. The most common test mixes sulfosalicylic acid with an equal amount of urine. The urine is first spun in a centrifuge to remove any particulate matter. Then it's mixed with the acid. The Hands On procedure on page 174 will guide you in performing this test.

If the strip test showed little or no protein, the urine-acid mixture in this confirmation test should remain clear. Cloudiness won't appear unless the urine contains at least 20 mg/dL of protein. The more protein in the urine, the cloudier the mixture will be.

BLOOD IN URINE

Small numbers of RBCs sometimes show up in urine. The kidneys have small blood vessels that normally don't allow blood to pass into the urine. However, blood can be present if the specimen has been contaminated by menstrual blood.

Hematuria also can be a sign of bleeding in the urinary tract. Such bleeding could result from:

- renal disorders
- a urinary tract infection (UTI)
- abnormal tissue growths or tumors
- trauma to the urinary tract
- kidney stones (calculi)

The reagent strip tests for blood in urine. The strip reacts to the hemoglobin found in red blood cells. However, the strip also reacts to myoglobin, a protein found in muscles.

Myoglobin may be released into the bloodstream because of over exercise, a crushing injury or other trauma, and some kinds of surgery. Then it's excreted in urine. So to avoid a false result, if the strip test is positive for blood, it should be confirmed by looking for RBCs under a microscope. If myoglobin is suspected, a specific test for it can be ordered.

MEASURING BILIRUBIN

Bilirubin is made when the body breaks down hemoglobin. It's processed in the liver before it's excreted into the intestines. High levels in urine can be a sign of:

- liver diseases such as hepatitis
- bile duct blockage in the liver
- destruction of red blood cells—for example, in a bad reaction to a blood transfusion

Bilirubin is another substance tested for on the reagent strip. However, its color can give urine an amber or dark yellow shade. This can make its pad on

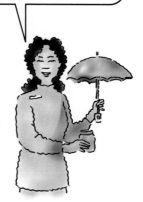

Test for bilirubin as soon as possible because it breaks down when exposed to light. Be sure to shield the specimen until you can do the test.

the test strip hard to read. Therefore, many labs confirm the result by using the diazo tablet method (Ictotest). You can learn how to do this test by following the Hands On procedure on page 176.

DETECTING UROBILINOGEN

After bilirubin is secreted into the intestines, bacteria there convert it into urobilinogen. Some of this chemical is absorbed through the intestines into the bloodstream. It's then excreted by the kidneys in urine. The rest passes through the intestines and leaves the body in feces.

Urobilinogen is detected in reagent strip testing. It's measured in Ehrlich units, a special measurement for urobilinogen. An Ehrlich unit is 1 mg/dL of urobilinogen. A value between 0.1 and 1.0 is considered normal. Any test result over 1.0 Ehrlich units/dL can be a warning sign. Here's what high levels of urobilinogen in urine can mean:

- a high rate of RBC destruction; this can result from the same things a high bilirubin level indicates.
- a bowel obstruction; if feces are forced to stay in the intestine, more urobilinogen will be reabsorbed into the blood and excreted by the kidneys in urine.
- a damaged liver; high urobilinogen levels can occur in the early stages of hepatitis or with other liver impairments.

NITRITE TESTING

Some bacteria that infect the urinary tract have an enzyme that changes the nitrates in urine to nitrites. In the nitrite test, urine is applied to the reagent pad. If the pad changes color, nitrites are present in the specimen.

A positive nitrite test signals that the patient has a UTI, or bacteriuria (bacteria in urine). However, if you delay for long in testing the urine, a small number of bacteria in it can multiply. A false-positive result for nitrites—and thus for a UTI—could occur. This is another good reason to get specimens to the lab quickly!

LEUKOCYTE ESTERASE

Leukocytes (WBCs) in the urine also mean that a UTI is present. Leukocytes called neutrophils enter the kidneys to fight infection. These neutrophils contain an enzyme called **esterase**. This is detected on a reagent strip that contains a leukocyte esterase reaction pad. Normal urine may contain a few white cells. Larger numbers must be present to produce a positive leukocyte esterase test.

Urine Sediment

Looking at a urine specimen under the microscope can confirm urinalysis results. It may also add more information that will help the physician diagnose the patient. However, microscopic examination of urine is not a CLIA-waived procedure. Unless your lab is CLIA-certified for higher-level tests, this work may be going to an outside lab.

If your lab is allowed to perform microscopy, you may be asked to prepare specimens for study. To prepare urine for a microscopic exam, the specimen must first be centrifuged. Here's what will happen next.

- The spinning forces the urine's particulate matter to the bottom of the test tube. This concentrates all the cells and other solids in one place as **sediment.** (Sediment is solid matter that settles to the bottom of a liquid.)

- This sediment is collected and suspended again in a much smaller amount of the **supernatant** urine (the top, liquid portion of spun urine).

- A drop of this more concentrated solution is placed on a slide for viewing under the microscope.

You'll find detailed instructions for preparing urine sediment for microscopy in the Hands On procedure on page 178.

Urine sediment is examined for:

- RBCs
- WBCs
- casts
- epithelial cells
- bacteria
- crystals

The illustrations on pages 157, 159, and 160 show you what each of these substances looks like under the microscope.

BLOOD CELLS

When the sediment contains red blood cells or RBCs, the strip test should also be positive for blood. As you've already read, RBCs in urine can mean a number of things.

Legal Brief URINE SEDIMENT EXAMS

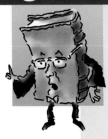

CLIA classifies urine sediment exams as moderate-complexity tests. Generally, a lab must have a Certificate of Compliance or Accreditation to perform tests at this level. However, CLIA allows other labs to examine urine sediment if they have a Certificate of Provider Performed Microscopy (PPM) Procedures. This certificate allows the following practitioners to perform PPM:

- physician (MD or DO)
- mid-level professional under a physician's supervision
- podiatrist
- dentist

There are other CLIA requirements for urine sediment testing.

- The lab must have written PPM procedures in place.
- A positive (abnormal results) control must be tested each day urine sediment is examined.
- The centrifuge and microscope must be cleaned and checked for accuracy regularly. Maintenance records must be kept for two years.

Sometimes, however, a microscopic exam won't find RBCs, even when the reagent strip test is positive. This can happen if the patient is suffering some kinds of hemolysis—for example, a transfusion reaction or a sickle cell crisis. (Remember that you read about sickle cell anemia in Chapter 3.)

As you also read earlier, a positive strip test result may occur if the patient's urine contains myoglobin. No red cells will be found in the urine sediment in this case either.

White blood cells (WBCs), or leukocytes, in the sediment can indicate a urinary tract infection. If they're present in large enough numbers, the leukocyte esterase test on the reagent strip will also be positive. The protein test on the strip may be positive too if some of the WBCs **lyse** (break apart). It will also be positive if the infection has reached the tubes of the kidneys.

If your lab is CLIA-certified, the physician might ask you to prepare urine sediment samples for study.

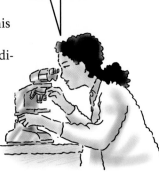

CELLS IN URINE

Epithelial Cells   Three types of epithelial cells may appear in urine sediment: renal tubular, transitional and/or squamous. Other types of cells may appear in urine but are difficult to identify due to morphologic changes caused by urine. Tubular cells are approximately ⅓ larger than white blood cells. Transitional epithelial cells may arise from the renal pelvis, ureters, bladder or urethra. They tend to be pear-shaped. Squamous cells are large and flat with a prominent nucleus. They originate in the urethra.

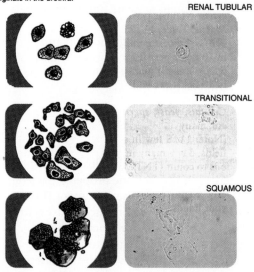

RENAL TUBULAR

TRANSITIONAL

SQUAMOUS

RBCs   Red blood cells may originate from any part of the renal system. The presence of large numbers of RBCs in the urine suggests infection, trauma, tumors, renal calculi, etc. However, the presence of 1 or 2 RBC/(HPF) in the urine sediment, or blood in the urine from menstrual contamination, should not be considered abnormal.

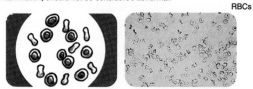

RBCs

WBCs   White blood cells in the urine (pyuria) may originate from any part of the renal system. The presence of more than 5 WBCs per HPF may suggest infection, cystitis, or pyelonephritis.

RENAL TUBULAR & WBC (SEDI-STAIN*)

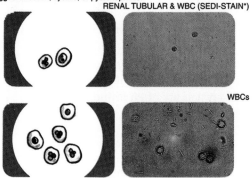

WBCs

Here are examples of cells found in urine sediment.

CASTS

Casts are cylinders of proteins and other substances that form and solidify in the nephron tubules in the kidneys. Most casts eventually break free and end up in the urine. Certain casts can indicate disease or infection. For example, in a kidney infection, WBCs become trapped in the protein network and form white cell casts.

Casts are examined using low-power magnification and reduced light. They provide good information about what's going on inside the kidneys' nephron tubules. They're reported as the number of casts counted within the microscope's low-power field.

BACTERIA AND CRYSTALS

Normal urine shouldn't contain bacteria if the clean-catch specimen was collected properly. If it wasn't done properly, bacteria on the skin could have been washed into the specimen. This would contaminate the sample and could produce a false result on the test strip. On the other hand, large amounts of bacteria in the urine can be a sign of a urinary tract infection.

As you've already read, the test strip relies on the nitrites produced by bacteria for a positive result. However, not all bacteria produce nitrites. Therefore, some kinds of bacteria may be found in urine sediment even when the strip test is negative.

Crystals appear when there are enough of certain chemicals in the urine to form solid structures. These structures are tiny, but they can be seen under the microscope. The following crystals are most commonly found in urine sediment.

- Calcium oxalate crystals can occur in urine that has a pH lower than 7.0.
- Uric acid crystals also may occur in urine with a pH lower than 7.0.
- Triple phosphate crystals can develop in urine with a pH above 7.0.

Crystals by themselves are not necessarily a problem. However, they can contribute to the formation of stones in the urinary tract. Also, uric acid crystals are often found in patients who have fever, leukemia, or gout.

EPITHELIAL CELLS

Epithelial cells cover the skin and organs, and line pathways like the digestive tract and urinary tract. Epithelial cells shed

CASTS IN URINE

Hyaline Casts   Hyaline casts are formed from a protein gel in the renal tubule. Hyaline casts may contain cellular inclusions. Hyaline casts will dissolve very rapidly in alkaline urine. Normal urine sediment may contain 1 to 2 hyaline casts per low power field (LPF).

HYALINE

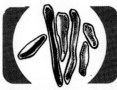 

Granular Casts   Granular casts are casts with granules present throughout the cast matrix. They are quite refractile. If the granules are small, the cast is defined as a finely granular cast. If granules are large, it is termed a coarsely granular cast. Granular casts can appear in urine in normal or abnormal states.

GRANULAR

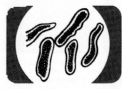 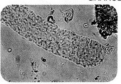

RBC Casts   RBC casts are pathologic and their presence is usually indicative of severe injury to the glomerulus. Rarely, transtubular bleeding may occur, forming RBC casts. RBC casts are found in acute glomerulonephritis, lupus, bacterial endocarditis and septicemias. "Blood" casts are granular and contain hemoglobin from degenerated RBCs.

RBC CASTS

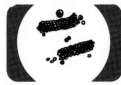 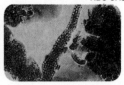

WBC Casts   WBC casts occur when leukocytes are incorporated within the cast matrix. WBC casts will usually indicate an infection, most commonly pyelonephritis. They may also be seen in glomerular diseases. WBC casts may be the only clue to pyelonephritis.

WBC CASTS

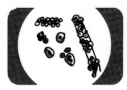 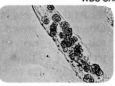

Here are examples of casts found in urine sediment.

CRYSTALS FOUND IN ACID URINE

URIC ACID (POLARIZED)

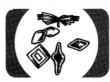 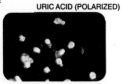

Leucine/Tyrosine Crystals Leucine and tyrosine are amino acids which crystallize and often appear together in the urine of patients with severe liver disease. Tyrosine usually appears as fine needles arranged as sheaves or rosettes and appear yellow. Leucine is usually yellow, oily-appearing spheres with radial and concentric striations.

TYROSINE (BRIGHTFIELD)

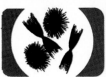 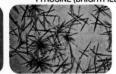

LEUCINE (BRIGHTFIELD)

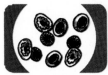 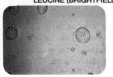

Cystine Crystals Cystine crystals are thin, hexagonal-shaped (6-sided) structures. They appear in the urine as a result of a genetic defect. Cystine crystals and stones will appear in the urine in cystinuria and homocystinuria. Cystine crystals are frequently confused with uric acid crystals. Cystine crystals do not polarize light.

CYSTINE (BRIGHTFIELD)

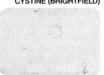

CYSTINE (POLARIZED)

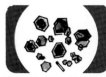 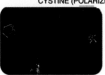

CRYSTALS FOUND IN ACID, NEUTRAL AND ALKALINE URINE
Calcium Oxalate Calcium oxalate crystals most frequently have an "envelope" shape and appear in acid, neutral or slightly alkaline urine. They appear in the urine after the ingestion of certain foods, i.e., cabbage, asparagus.

CALCIUM OXALATE (BRIGHTFIELD)

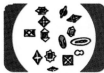 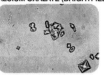

Hippuric Acid Hippuric acid crystals are colorless or pale yellow. They occur as needles, six-sided prisms, or star-shaped clusters. They appear in urine after the ingestion of certain vegetables and fruits with benzoic acid content. They have little clinical significance.

HIPPURIC ACID (BRIGHTFIELD)

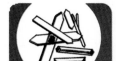 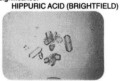

CRYSTALS FOUND IN ACID URINE
Uric Acid Crystals Uric acid has birefringent characteristics; therefore, it polarizes light, giving multi-colors. Uric acid crystals are found in acid urine. Uric acid may assume various forms, e.g., rhombic, plates, rosettes, small crystals. The color may be red-brown, yellow or colorless. Although increased in 16% of patients with gout, and in patients with malignant lymphoma or leukemia, their presence does not usually indicate pathology or increased uric acid concentrations.

URIC ACID (BRIGHTFIELD)

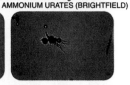

CRYSTALS FOUND IN ALKALINE URINE
Ammonium Biurate or Ammonium Urates Ammonium urates are yellow-brown in appearance and occur in urine as spheres or spheres with spicules ("thorny apples"). Both forms are frequently seen together. They appear in urine when there is ammonia formation in the urine present in the bladder. They are considered to have little clinical significance.

AMMONIUM URATES (BRIGHTFIELD)

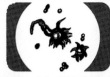 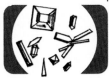

Triple Phosphate Triple phosphate crystals are common in urine sediment. They have a "coffin-lid" shape, are colorless and appear in alkaline urine. The ingestion of fruit may cause triple phosphate to appear in urine.

TRIPLE PHOSPHATE (BRIGHTFIELD)

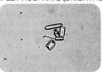

Here are examples of crystals found in urine sediment.

and are normally found in urine, but a large number in a specimen can be a sign of inflammation somewhere in the urinary system.

Three types of epithelial cells may be found in urine.

- Squamous epithelial cells cover the body's outer skin surfaces. They are a normal finding in urine because the urine comes in contact with the skin during urination.
- Transitional epithelial cells line the bladder. They show up in urine in cystitis and other infections of the lower urinary tract.
- Renal epithelial cells line the nephrons of the kidneys. They're seen with infections and inflammations of the upper urinary tract.

There's no chemical test for epithelial cells. They can be seen in urine sediment, however. When renal epithelial cells are seen, it's likely that the renal tubules have been damaged. Also, the strip test for protein may be positive if these cells are present.

OTHER STRUCTURES

Other things also can be found in urine sediment. For example, a patient with a vaginal yeast infection can contaminate her specimen with yeast. Yeast also can appear in urine if the patient has a UTI. This is especially true of diabetic patients.

The parasite *Trichomonas vaginalis* can contaminate urine from the genital tract of an infected person. Mucus can be present in the sediment if the patient's urinary tract is inflamed. Mucus threads are usually reported as *few*, *moderate*, or *many* in number. Sperm may be found in the urine of a male patient who has recently ejaculated.

Urine Testing for Pregnancy

You first read about pregnancy tests in Chapter 4. They look for the presence of human chorionic gonadotropin (HCG) in the woman's urine or serum. HCG is a hormone that is secreted by the developing placenta shortly after conception takes place.

Most urine pregnancy test kits are easy to use. You simply add urine to the test and read the result. All pregnancy tests measure some part of the HCG molecule. They can detect tiny levels of HCG in urine just 10 to 12 days after conception. This is sometimes even before a woman's first missed period.

Some of the newer pregnancy test kits use ELISA, which you also read about in Chapter 4. ELISA pregnancy tests use an antibody that's specific for one site on the HCG molecule. Another reagent antibody seeks a second site on the molecule. When the HCG antigen is present in urine or serum, a reaction occurs and the test changes color.

When using urine in a pregnancy test, a first-morning urine sample is best. Urine is most concentrated in the morning, which makes the hormone easier to detect. Most labs also do a specific gravity test along with the pregnancy test. If the specimen's specific gravity is below 1.015, they won't report a negative result on the pregnancy test. That's because the urine may be too dilute to detect low levels of HCG.

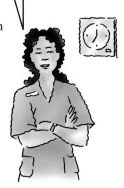

When performing a pregnancy test, it's best to use the first urine of the day because it's the most concentrated.

Urine Drug Testing

To test urine for drugs, your lab must use a commercial test approved by the U.S. Food and Drug Administration (FDA). In addition, the patient must test positive for a drug on two separate tests before you can report a positive result. Either of the following test outcomes will result in a negative finding:

- The specimen contains no drug.
- The drug's concentration is below the level required for a positive result.

If the first test comes up negative, no further testing is done. If that test result is positive, a confirming test is performed. A method called gas chromatography/mass spectrometry (GC/MS) is used in confirmation testing for drugs.

Here are some of the drugs that can be detected in urine:

- amphetamines
- barbiturates
- benzodiazepines
- cocaine
- marijuana
- methadone
- opioids
- PCP

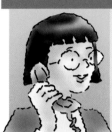

Ask the Professional   DRUG TEST RESULTS

Q: *Our office gives preemployment physicals for several employers in the area. Patients sometimes ask if the results of the drug screen that's part of the physical exam are confidential. How should I answer such questions?*

A: Under most circumstances, the results of a blood or urine test are part of a patient's private medical record. However, if the exam is being paid for by the employer, the company must be provided with all the results.

Assure the patient that his medical records will be kept as confidential as possible. Also, tell him that since this is a preemployment physical, the employer will get all the results of this exam. Remind the patient that he has a right to refuse the urine drug test, but also note that the employer may require a negative drug screen as a condition of employment.

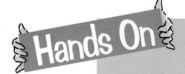

OBTAINING A CLEAN-CATCH MIDSTREAM URINE SPECIMEN

5-1

Follow these steps to instruct patients how to collect a clean-catch midstream urine specimen.

1. Gather your equipment. To obtain a clean-catch midstream urine specimen, you'll need the following: a clean, dry (or sterile) urine container labeled with the patient's name; antiseptic wipes; a bedpan or urinal (if necessary); and gloves (if you'll be assisting the patient).

2. Wash your hands. Put on gloves if you'll be assisting the patient.

3. Greet and identify the patient. Explain the procedure. Ask for and answer any questions the patient may have.

4. If the patient will perform the procedure, give the patient the proper supplies.

5. Tell patients that they must follow the procedure exactly or the specimen may be contaminated and produce false test results. Also, keep in mind that many patients might not know what the meatus or glans labia are, so be sure to explain in your instructions if necessary.

6. Instruct male patients:
   - Wash your hands upon entering the bathroom. Remove the lid from the container and place the lid flat side down in the designated area. Be careful not to touch the inside of the lid.
   - If uncircumcised, retract the foreskin to expose the glans penis. Clean the meatus with an antiseptic wipe. Use a new wipe for each cleaning sweep.
   - Keep the foreskin retracted and void for a second into the toilet or urinal. It's important to do this first so the specimen will have the least contamination with the skin.
   - While maintaining a stream, bring the sterile container into the urine stream. Collect 30 to 100 mL. Don't touch the inside of the container with the penis.
   - Once a sufficient amount has been collected, finish voiding into the toilet or urinal.
   - Cap the specimen container and wash your hands. Bring the container to the designated area.

   Test, transfer, or store the container according to your office's policy.

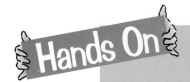

OBTAINING A CLEAN-CATCH MIDSTREAM URINE SPECIMEN (*continued*)   **5-1**

7. Instruct female patients:
   - Wash your hands upon entering the bathroom. Remove the lid from the container and place the lid flat side down in the designated area. Be careful not to touch the inside of the lid.
   - Kneel or squat over a bedpan or toilet. Spread the labia minora to expose the meatus. First, cleanse on each side of the meatus. Wipe from front to back, using a new wipe for each side. Then, using a new wipe, clean the meatus itself. Again, wipe from front to back.
   - Keeping the labia separated, initially void for a second into the toilet or bedpan. It's important to do this first so the specimen will have the least contamination with the skin.
   - While maintaining a stream, bring the sterile container into the stream and collect 30 to 100 mL.
   - Once a sufficient amount has been collected, finish voiding into the toilet or bedpan.
   - Cap the specimen container and wash your hands. Bring the container to the designated area.

   Test, transfer, or store the container according to your office's policy.

8. Use gloves when handling the specimen container returned by the patient. Then clean the work area, remove your gloves, and wash your hands.

9. Record the procedure.

Hands On

PERFORMING A CHEMICAL REAGENT STRIP ANALYSIS

5-2

Follow these steps to perform a reagent strip test (dipstick test) to screen chemical properties of a urine specimen.

1. Wash your hands.

2. Assemble the equipment: a chemical strip (such as Multistix or Chemstrip), the manufacturer's color comparison chart, a stopwatch or timer, a 15 × 125 mm test tube or Kova system urine tube, and a patient report form or data form.

3. Put on an impervious gown, a face shield, and gloves.

4. Verify that the names on the specimen container and the report form are the same.

5. Mix the patient's urine by gently swirling the specimen container. Then pour 12 mL of urine into a Kova system urine tube.

6. Remove a reagent strip from its container and replace the lid to prevent deterioration of the strips by humidity. Don't remove the desiccant package from the container. It keeps moisture levels in the container to a minimum.

7. Immerse the reagent strip in the urine completely, then immediately remove it, sliding the edge of the strip along the lip of the tube to remove excess urine. Turn the strip on its edge and touch the edge to a paper towel or other absorbent paper. Immediate removal and touching its edge to a paper towel prevents colors from leaching due to prolonged exposure to urine.

8. Start your stopwatch or timer immediately after removing the strip from the urine. Reactions must be read at specific times as directed in the package insert and on the color comparison chart.

9. Compare the reagent pads to the color chart. Determine the results at intervals stated by the test strip manufacturer.
   - Example: Glucose is read at 30 seconds. For that result, examine the glucose pad 30 seconds after dipping and compare it with the color chart for glucose.

10. Read all the reactions at the times indicated and record the results.

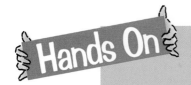

PERFORMING A CHEMICAL REAGENT STRIP ANALYSIS (*continued*)

5-2

11. Discard the used strip in a biohazard container. Discard the urine in accordance with your office's policies.

12. Properly care for or dispose of equipment and supplies. Clean the work area using a ten-percent bleach solution. Remove your gown, face shield, and gloves. Then wash your hands.

Precautions for chemical strip testing:

- False-positive and false-negative results are possible. Review the manufacturer's package insert to learn about factors that may give false results and how to avoid them.

- If the patient is taking Pyridium, don't use a reagent strip for testing because the medication will interfere with the color.

- Outdated materials give inaccurate results. If the strip's expiration date has passed, discard it.

Hands On

DETERMINING THE COLOR AND CLARITY OF URINE

5-3

Follow these steps to determine the color and clarity of a urine specimen. Note that some urine turns cloudy if left standing. Color and clarity must be determined rapidly.

1. Wash your hands.

2. Assemble the equipment: a clear test tube, a sheet of white paper with scored black lines, and a patient report form or data form.

3. Put on gloves, an impervious gown, and a face shield.

4. Verify that the names on the specimen container and the report form are the same.

5. Pour 10 to 15 mL of urine from the container into the test tube.

6. In a bright light against a white background, examine the color of the urine in the tube.
   - The intensity of yellow color, which is due to urochrome, depends on urine concentration.
   - The most common colors are straw (very pale yellow), yellow, and dark yellow.

7. Determine clarity by holding the tube in front of the white paper scored with black lines.
   - If you can see the lines clearly, record the sample as clear.
   - If the lines are not well defined when viewed through the sample, record it as hazy.
   - If you can't see the lines at all through the sample, record it as cloudy.

8. If further testing is to be done but will be delayed more than an hour, refrigerate the specimen to avoid chemical changes.

9. Properly care for or dispose of equipment and supplies. Clean the work area using a ten-percent bleach solution. Remove your gown, face shield, and gloves. Then wash your hands.

Charting Example:
05/31/2007 2:45 P.M. Random urine collected. Yellow/clear.
_____ H. Henderson, RMA

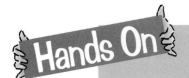

**PERFORMING A CLINITEST
FOR REDUCING SUGARS**

5-4

Follow these steps to perform a Clinitest. This may be used as a confirming test for glucose when reagent strips test in a trace value or greater, or can't be interpreted. It's also used to test children under age two for inborn errors of metabolism, regardless of the glucose strip test result.

1. Wash your hands.

2. Assemble the equipment: transfer pipettes, distilled water, positive and negative controls, a stopwatch or timer, a Clinitest color comparison chart, Clinitest tablets, a daily sample log, 16×125 mm glass test tubes, a test tube rack, and a patient report form or data form.

3. Put on an impervious gown, a face shield, and gloves.

4. Identify the specimen to be tested and record patient and sample information in the daily log.

5. Record on the report or data form the patient's identification information, catalog and lot numbers for all test and control materials, and expiration dates. This is required by CLIA regulations and QA/QC procedures.

6. Label test tubes with patient and control identification and put them in the test tube rack.

7. Using a transfer pipette, add ten drops of distilled water to each labeled test tube in the rack. Hold the dropper vertically to ensure proper delivery of the drops into the tube.

8. Add five drops of the patient's urine or five drops of control sample to each tube, according to its label (for example, positive control sample to the tube labeled *positive control* and so on). Use a different transfer pipette for each tube. This prevents contaminating any of the samples.

9. Open the Clinitest bottle and shake a tablet into the lid without touching it. Then drop the tablet from the lid into the test tube. Repeat for all patient and control samples being tested. Close the Clinitest bottle.
   - Touching the tablet may cause false results.
   - The Clinitest bottle must be kept tightly capped at all times because moisture causes the tablets to deteriorate. This will affect test results.

(continued)

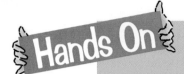

**PERFORMING A CLINITEST
FOR REDUCING SUGARS (*continued*)**

5-4

10. Observe reactions in the test tubes as the mixture boils. After the reaction stops, wait 15 seconds, then gently swirl the test tubes. This mixes the contents so you can read the results.
    • Watch carefully during the boiling to see if the contents of the patient's tube pass through all the colors on the five-drop color chart before ending in a final color.
    • If this happens, the test result should be reported as "exceeds 2%."
    • If your lab requires a more exact result on this pass-through reaction, perform the two-drop method according to the Clinitest package insert and use the two-drop color chart for interpretation.

11. Immediately compare results for the patient specimen and the controls with the five-drop method color chart (see example on p. 171).
    • The positive and negative controls ensure testing accuracy.
    • If the positive and negative controls don't give expected results, the test is invalid and must be repeated.
    • Certain medications (for example, ascorbic acid) and reducing substances other than glucose (galactose and lactose) may cause false-positive results. If this occurs, further testing is necessary.

12. Properly care for or dispose of equipment and supplies. Clean the work area using a ten-percent bleach solution. Remove your gown, face shield, and gloves. Then wash your hands.

Charting Example:
04/21/2007 9:00 A.M. Random urine tested for glucose.
Clinitest, results ¾%. _____ N. Peterson, RMA

5-Drop Method Standard Procedure

DIRECTIONS FOR TESTING:

1. Collect urine in clean container. With dropper in upright position, place **5 drops** of urine in test tube. Rinse dropper with water and add 10 drops of water to test tube.

2. Drop one tablet into test tube. Watch while complete boiling reaction takes place. Do not shake test tube during boiling, or for the following 15 seconds after boiling has stopped.
3. At the end of this 15-second waiting period, shake test tube gently to mix contents. Compare

color of liquid to Color Chart below. Ignore sediment that may form in the bottom of the test tube. Ignore changes after the 15-second waiting period.
4. Write down the percent (%) result which appears on the color block that most closely matches the color of the liquid.

NEGATIVE	1/4%	1/2%	3/4%	1%	2% or more

Here's an example of a Clinitest package insert.

Hands On

PERFORMING A NITROPRUSSIDE REACTION (ACETEST) FOR KETONES

5-5

Follow these steps to perform this confirmation test to determine the level of ketones in urine.

1. Wash your hands.

2. Assemble the equipment: white filter paper, a plastic transfer pipette, an ACETEST tablet, the manufacturer's color comparison chart, a stopwatch or timer that displays time to the second, and a patient report form or data form.

3. Put on an impervious gown, a face shield, and gloves.

4. Identify the specimen to be tested and record patient and sample information in the daily log.

5. Record on the report or data form the patient's identification information, catalog and lot numbers for all test and control materials, and expiration dates. This is required by CLIA regulations and QA/QC procedures.

6. Shake an ACETEST tablet into the cap and put it on the filter paper. Replace the cap.
   - Dispensing the tablet in this manner prevents contamination of the tablet or the bottle's contents.
   - The white background of the filter paper provides contrast for the test results.

7. Using a transfer pipette, place one drop of urine on top of the tablet.

8. Wait 30 seconds for the complete reaction. A reaction will occur if ketones are present in the urine.

9. Compare the color of the tablet to the manufacturer's color chart (see example on p. 173). Record the results as negative, small amount, moderate amount, or large amount.

10. Properly care for or dispose of equipment and supplies. Clean the work area using a ten-percent bleach solution. Remove your gown, face shield, and gloves. Then wash your hands.

Charting Example:
11/20/2007 8:00 A.M. Urine specimen collected and tested for ketones; results showed large amount. Dr. Wendt notified.

_____ B. Evans, CMA

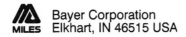

Bayer Corporation
Elkhart, IN 46515 USA

Colors shown below are for use with ACETEST Reagent Tablets only.

NEGATIVE   **SMALL**   **MODERATE**   **LARGE**

Here's an example of an ACETEST package insert.

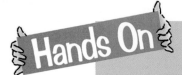

PERFORMING AN ACID PRECIPITATION TEST FOR PROTEIN

5-6

Follow these steps to perform this confirmation test for determining the level of protein in urine.

1. Wash your hands.

2. Assemble the equipment: a test tube rack, clear test tubes, transfer pipettes, positive and negative controls, a stopwatch or timer, a daily sample log, three-percent sulfosalicylic acid (SSA) solution, and a patient report form or data form.

3. Put on an impervious gown, a face shield, and gloves.

4. Identify the patient's specimen to be tested, and record patient and sample information on the daily log. This step prevents errors and fulfills QA/QC requirements.

5. Record on the report or data form the patient's name or identification, catalog and lot numbers for all test and control materials, and expiration dates. This step fulfills QA/QC requirements.

6. Label the test tubes with patient and control identification. Then place them in the test tube rack.

7. Centrifuge the patient sample at 1,500 rpm for five minutes.

8. Add one to three mL of supernatant urine or control sample to the patient and control-labeled tubes in the rack. Use a clean transfer pipette for each.

9. Add an equal amount of three-percent SSA to the sample quantity in each tube.

10. Mix the contents of the tubes and let them stand for two to ten minutes. Use a stopwatch or timer to make sure you perform the next step within this time frame.

11. Mix the contents of the tubes again, then observe the degree of turbidity in each test tube. Assign a score according to the following guidelines.
    - neg: no turbidity or cloudiness; urine remains clear
    - trace: slight turbidity
    - 1+: turbidity with no precipitation
    - 2+: heavy turbidity with fine granulation
    - 3+: heavy turbidity with granulation and flakes
    - 4+: clumps of precipitated protein

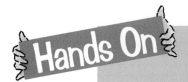

PERFORMING AN ACID PRECIPITATION TEST FOR PROTEIN (*continued*)

5-6

12. The specimen may be matched against a McFarland standard for objective assessment. If positive and negative controls don't give the expected results, the test is invalid and must be repeated.

13. Properly care for or dispose of equipment and supplies. Clean the work area using a ten-percent bleach solution. Remove your gown, face shield, and gloves. Then wash your hands.

Charting Example:
03/28/2007 9:00 A.M. Urine specimen collected and tested for protein; results 3+ using acid precipitation test.

_____ R. McDonald, CMA

Hands On

PERFORMING THE DIAZO TABLET TEST (ICTOTEST) FOR BILIRUBIN

5-7

Follow these steps to perform a diazo tablet test for bilirubin. Note that the specimen must be free of Pyridium, chlorpromazine, and other drugs that interfere with color interpretation.

1. Wash your hands.
2. Assemble the equipment: Ictotest white mats, a stopwatch or timer, a transfer pipette, diazo (Ictotest) tablets, a clean paper towel, and a patient report form or data form.
3. Put on an impervious gown, a face shield, and gloves.
4. Verify that the names on the specimen container and the report form are the same.
5. Place the Ictotest white mat on a clean, dry paper towel.
   - The mat provides a testing surface.
   - The paper towel must be dry because moisture may cause a false result.
6. Using a clean transfer pipette, add ten drops of urine to the center of the mat.
   - If the urine is red, it may be difficult to read the reaction properly. In this case, pour an aliquot of the urine into a urine tube or test tube.
   - Centrifuge as if preparing urine sediment. (See the following Hands On procedure.) Use ten drops of the supernatant in this step.
7. Shake a diazo tablet into the bottle cap and put it into the center of the mat. Do not touch the tablet. Touching it contaminates it and could cause a false-positive result.
8. Recap the bottle immediately to prevent the other tablets from deteriorating. The tablets must be protected from exposure to light, heat, and moisture.
9. Use a clean transfer pipette to place one drop of water on the tablet. Then wait five seconds.
10. Add another drop of water to the tablet so that the solution formed by the first drop runs onto the mat. This lets the diazo chemical react with the urine.

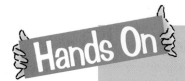

**PERFORMING THE DIAZO
TABLET TEST (ICTOTEST)
FOR BILIRUBIN** (*continued*)

5-7

11. Within 60 seconds, observe for color on the mat around the tablet.
    - A blue or purple color indicates a positive result for bilirubin.
    - A pink or red color indicates a negative result.

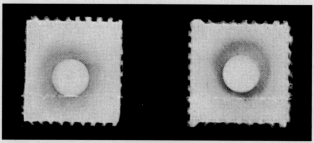

Here are examples of negative (left) and positive (right) test results from an Ictotest package insert.

12. Properly care for or dispose of equipment and supplies. Clean the work area using a ten-percent bleach solution. Remove your gown, face shield, and gloves. Then wash your hands.

Charting Example:
3/23/2007 9:30 A.M. Urine specimens collected and tested for bilirubin using diazo testing. Results positive.

_____ K. Rogers, CMA

Hands On

PREPARING URINE SEDIMENT 5-8

Follow these steps to prepare a urine sediment sample for microscopic examination. Note that if the specimen is to be tested by chemical reagent strip, this can be done before or after centrifuging the urine.

1. Wash your hands.
2. Assemble the equipment: a centrifuge, urine centrifuge tubes, a transfer pipette, and a patient report form or data form.
3. Put on an impervious gown, a face shield, and gloves.
4. Verify that the names on the specimen container and the report form are the same.
5. Swirl the specimen to mix. Pour 10 or 12 mL of well-mixed urine into a labeled urine centrifuge tube or a tube provided by the test system manufacturer. Cap the tube with a plastic cap or parafilm.
   - Some test systems use 10 mL and some use 12 mL. The 12 mL volume allows reagent strip testing from the same tube. Check your lab procedures to find out which type of tube to use.
   - Some patients cannot produce a large amount of urine. If less than the standard 10 or 12 mL of urine is available, document the actual volume prepared on the report form. This is necessary to ensure proper interpretation of results.
   - Preparing a urine sediment sample from less than three mL of specimen is not recommended.
6. Centrifuge the sample at 1,500 rpm for five minutes. This ensures that cellular and particulate matter is pulled to the bottom of the tube.
7. When the centrifuge has stopped, remove the tubes. After making sure no tests are to be performed first on the supernatant, pour off all but 0.5 to 1.0 mL of it. Follow the manufacturer's directions for this procedure.
8. Suspend the sediment again in the remaining supernatant by aspirating up into the bulbous portion of a urine transfer pipette.
9. Place a urine slide (Kova slide or other urine system slide) on the counter. Add a drop of the mixed sediment on the

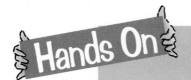

PREPARING URINE SEDIMENT (*continued*)

5-8

slide with built in coverslip (follow the test system's manufacturer's directions for doing this). The concentrated urine is now prepared for microscopic examination.

10. Properly care for or dispose of equipment and supplies. Clean the work area using a ten-percent bleach solution. Remove your gown, face shield, and gloves. Then wash your hands.

Note: Centrifuge maintenance requires regular checks to ensure that the timing and speed are correct. Document this information on the maintenance log.

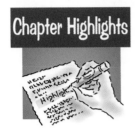

Chapter Highlights

- Urinalysis helps the physician determine or rule out conditions to make a correct diagnosis.

- The medical assistant's role is to assist in the collection of uncontaminated specimens and to perform reagent strip screening and confirmation tests on patients' urine.

- Clean-catch midstream urine collection is the most common method for collecting a urine specimen.

- Physical examination of urine includes observation of color and clarity and measuring specific gravity.

- Chemical tests include determining the urine's pH and checking for glucose, ketones, proteins, blood, bilirubin, urobilinogen, nitrites, and leukocytes in the specimen.

- Medical assistants also may prepare specimens for urine sediment exams.

- Urine sediment is examined under a microscope by a highly trained professional for things such as blood cells and casts, epithelial cells, bacteria, crystals, and other structures.

- Urine also may be tested to determine pregnancy and the presence of certain drugs in the body.

Chapter 6

CLINICAL CHEMISTRY

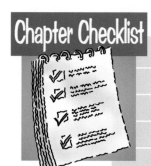

Chapter Checklist

- Explain the purpose of performing clinical chemistry tests
- List the common panels of chemistry tests
- List the instruments used for chemical testing
- List tests used to evaluate renal function
- List the common electrolytes and explain the relationship of electrolytes to body function
- Describe the nonprotein nitrogenous compounds and name conditions associated with abnormal values
- Describe the substances commonly tested in liver function assessment
- Explain thyroid function and identify the hormone that regulates the thyroid gland
- Describe how laboratory tests help assess for a myocardial infarction
- Describe how pancreatitis is diagnosed with laboratory tests
- Explain how the body uses and regulates glucose and summarize the purpose of the major glucose tests
- Determine a patient's blood glucose level
- Perform glucose tolerance testing
- Describe the function of cholesterol and other lipids and their correlation to heart disease

Blood chemistry tests measure important substances in the body. These tests are a valuable tool in helping physicians assess a patient's state of health. Although most chemistry tests are referred to outside labs for processing, this testing increasingly is being done in physician office labs. Several chemistry tests are CLIA-waived and can therefore be performed by medical assistants.

No matter where the chemistry tests ordered in your office are performed, you need to have a good general knowledge of these important tests and what their results can mean. In this chapter, you'll learn the basic principles of clinical chemistry testing.

Clinical Chemistry: Scope and Purpose

Clinical chemistry is just what the term suggests it is—laboratory testing for many of the chemical substances found in the body. This is determined by analyzing the following fluids:

- serum
- plasma
- whole blood
- other body fluids—that is, fluids that collect in the body's cavities

The chemical substances found in these fluids exist in several different forms. These include:

- electrically charged atoms called **ions;** ions are chemical elements that carry an electrical charge. For example, K^+, Na^+, and Cl^- are ions of the elements potassium, sodium, and chlorine, respectively.
- byproducts of the body's metabolic processes, for example, urea and creatinine
- proteins such as albumin and globulin
- hormones including testosterone and thyroid-stimulating hormone (TSH)

STUDYING CHEMICAL SUBSTANCES

Knowing the amount of various chemical substances in the body helps the physician in two ways.

- It helps the physician assess the function of certain organs. For example, knowing the level of bilirubin in a patient's blood helps show how well the patient's liver is functioning.

- It helps the physician gain a better understanding of the patient's overall health status. For example, knowing a patient's glucose and cholesterol levels can help the physician evaluate the patient's health.

TESTS AND TESTING METHODS

A large number of chemistry tests can be performed using blood collected either by venipuncture or skin puncture. Many of these tests are grouped according to body system. These groups of tests are called panels or profiles. Panels of chemistry tests can evaluate:

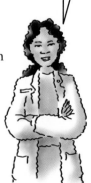

Specimen collection, reporting, and follow-up of patient care are critical aspects of your role as a medical assistant. This information directly impacts the patient's treatment and recovery.

- renal function
- liver function
- thyroid function
- cardiac function
- pancreatic function
- levels of lipids and lipoproteins

Only a few specific tests are performed in the physician office lab (POL). Because most chemistry panels aren't performed there, this chapter won't describe them in great detail. However, you must have a basic understanding of them so that you can take lab reports by phone. You should know what abnormal results may mean for the patient. Plus, you must understand the purpose of those chemistry tests that *are* conducted in the POL.

The table on page 207 summarizes the most common chemistry panel tests, the normal range for each test, and possible reasons for abnormal results. You'll find more information throughout this chapter about each of the tests listed in the table.

INSTRUMENTS AND METHODS OF TESTING

The spectrophotometer is still widely used for measuring various substances in a patient's blood. When certain chemical substances react with other chemicals, a color formation or a color change results. By measuring the change in the intensity of the color, the concentration of the substance can be determined.

Reference laboratories use automated systems to perform much of the chemical analysis. These systems mechanically sample, dilute, or add reagents (chemicals) to the patient's blood to measure the chemical substances in it. Automation has many benefits, including:

- fast test results
- less operator error
- controlled testing costs because of less need for human involvement

Remember, the normal ranges for results stated in this chapter may vary from lab to lab because different substrates (the substances on which a chemical acts), temperatures, and instruments may be used in testing.

Tests for Renal Function

The kidneys rid the body of waste products. They also help maintain fluid balance and acid-base balance. Acid-base balance is the balance between acid and base, or alkalis, in the body.

When the kidneys begin to fail, waste products, such as urea, ammonia, and creatinine, build up in the blood. As a result, the patient may develop **edema** (swelling due to excess fluid), and the delicate acid-base balance is upset. Abnormal increases or decreases in the substances that affect acid-base balance can harm a patient's health. In some cases, the patient could die.

The physician evaluates renal or kidney function by ordering tests to measure levels of electrolytes, blood urea nitrogen (BUN), creatinine, and uric acid. Based on the results of these tests, along with urinalysis, the physician can assess renal func-

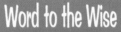

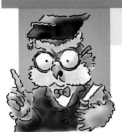

spectrophotometer (SPEK-tro-fo-TOM-ih-tuhr)

an instrument that measures light in a solution to determine the concentration of substances in it

tion. (For more information about chemistry tests that evaluate renal function, see the table on page 207.)

ELECTROLYTES

Electrolytes are ions in blood and body fluids. Remember, ions are chemicals that carry an electrical charge. Ions may have a positive charge or a negative charge. Positively charged ions are called **cations**. Negatively charged ions are known as **anions**.

The electrolytes found in the blood include:

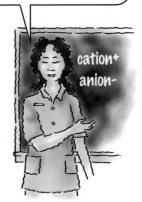

Remember, a _cation_ is a positively charged ion, and an _anion_ is a negatively charged ion. Both are electrolytes.

cation+
anion-

- sodium
- potassium
- chloride
- calcium
- magnesium
- phosphorus
- **bicarbonate** (dissolved carbon dioxide)

The renal system helps regulate electrolytes as well as fluid and acid-base balance. If the electrolytes are out of balance, the electrical impulses aren't passed on properly. The results are fluid and acid-base imbalances and poor functioning of the nervous and muscle tissue.

Sodium

Sodium is the major cation of the body's **extracellular fluid** (the fluid outside the cell). Its chemical symbol is Na.

Normal serum levels of sodium range from 135 to 145 mEq/L. When levels are below 135 mEq/L, the patient has a condition called hyponatremia. This is one of the most common electrolyte imbalances. Hyponatremia can result from many things:

- gastrointestinal losses (vomiting and diarrhea)
- severe burns
- cardiac failure
- renal failure
- hypothyroidism (underactive thyroid)

Symptoms of hyponatremia vary depending on how severe the condition is but may include changes in energy levels and seizures.

Hypernatremia occurs when a patient's sodium levels are above 145 mEq/L. Drug therapy, Cushing's syndrome, and diabetes insipidus are among the causes of hypernatremia.

Potassium

Potassium is the major cation of the body's **intracellular fluid** (the fluid inside the cell). Its chemical symbol is K. Because only two percent of potassium is extracellular, its serum levels are much lower (3.5 to 5.0 mEq/L) than sodium's serum levels. Abnormal levels of potassium in the blood can cause:

- muscle weakness
- paralysis
- cardiac arrhythmias (abnormal heart rhythms)

A serum potassium level below 3.5 mEq/L is called hypokalemia. This condition can occur because of:

- insulin therapy
- gastrointestinal losses
- renal disease

When a patient's potassium level is above 5.0 mEq/L, the result is known as hyperkalemia. Abnormally high potassium levels can be caused by:

- cell injuries
- renal failure

In addition, artifactual (caused by an outside interference) hyperkalemia can result from a traumatic venipuncture, hemolysis of red blood cells (RBCs), or if the tourniquet is on the patient's arm too long or too tightly when blood is being drawn.

INTRACELLULAR AND EXTRACELLULAR

Remember, *intracellular* fluid is fluid *inside* the cells. *Extracellular* fluid is fluid *outside* the cells. Electrolytes exist in both intracellular and extracellular fluid.

Chloride

Chloride is the major anion of the extracellular fluid. Its chemical symbol is Cl^-. The normal range for chloride is 96 to 110 mEq/L. Chloride is closely connected with the body's acid-base balance. In conditions such as diabetic ketoacidosis (high blood glucose caused by a lack of insulin) and metabolic acidosis (increased metabolic acids), a patient's chloride level can become abnormal.

The body normally loses chloride in urine, sweat, and stomach secretions. However, a serum chloride level that drops below 96 mEq/L is known as hypochloremia. This condition can occur from heavy sweating, vomiting, and renal failure, as well as several other conditions or diseases. Extremely low chloride levels can be fatal to a patient.

A patient with a serum chloride level above 110 MEq/L has a condition known as hyperchloremia. Dehydration and diarrhea also can cause this condition, as can a number of medications and gastrointestinal and metabolic problems.

Calcium

Calcium is another cation. Its chemical symbol is Ca. Normal Ca levels in blood range from 8.5 to 10.5 mg/dL.

Serum calcium levels significantly below 8.5 mg/dL are known as hypocalcemia. This condition can occur as a result of acute or chronic renal failure or electrolyte imbalance due to hypoparathyroidism.

Patients with hypercalcemia have calcium levels that are above 10.5 mg/dL. Hypercalcemia can occur in a patient with hyperparathyroidism. It also can occur if a patient has absorbed excessive amounts of calcium because of a medication he is taking or because of a change in gastrointestinal metabolism.

Cardiac arrhythmia may be a symptom of either hypomagnesemia or hypermagnesemia.

Magnesium

Magnesium is a cation found in intracellular fluid. Its chemical symbol is Mg, and its normal levels in blood are from 1.3 to 2.1 mEq/L. Hypomagnesemia occurs when a patient's serum magnesium level is below 1.3 mEq/L. This condition may result from shifts in body fluids and other electrolytes.

Hypermagnesemia, or serum magnesium levels above 2.1 mEq/L, also can result from fluid and electrolyte shifts, as well as from impaired excretion of fluids caused by kidney failure. The symptoms of hypermagnesemia and hyperkalemia (high levels of serum potassium) are similar.

Phosphorus

In the intracellular fluid, phosphorus is a major anion. Its chemical symbol is P. The normal range for phosphorus levels in blood is from 2.5 to 4.5 mg/dL. Hypophosphatemia (phosphorus levels below 2.5 mg/dL) can occur in patients for a number of reasons, including:

- inadequate absorption by the intestines of phosphorus consumed in food
- gastrointestinal losses, for example, through severe diarrhea

- electrolyte shifts between the blood and cells
- endocrine disorders (You'll read more about the endocrine system later in this chapter.)
- the withdrawal process from alcohol abuse

Hyperphosphatemia (serum phosphorus levels above 4.5 mg/dL) can happen when patients experience:

- hypocalcemia
- hypoparathyroidism
- renal damage or failure

In patients with renal failure, soft tissue calcification (hardening) is a long-term effect of hyperphosphatemia.

Bicarbonate

In the blood, bicarbonate (chemical symbol HCO_3) occurs when carbon dioxide dissolves in the bloodstream. The bicarbonate forms another negatively charged ion in the extracellular fluid. The normal bicarbonate range is 22 to 29 mmoles/L of total CO_2. Bicarbonate plays a major role in the delicate acid-base balance. If bicarbonate levels are increased, the patient develops **alkalosis** (the body pH is too basic, or alkaline). If bicarbonate levels are decreased, the patient develops **acidosis** (the body pH is too acidic).

As you've already read, the acid-base balance in the body is very sensitive. The body can't tolerate large changes in pH. Normally, its pH range is 7.35 to 7.45, which is slightly basic. (A neutral pH—neither acidic nor alkaline—is 7.0.)

Together, the renal and respiratory systems work to regulate the body's acid-base balance. Here's how they do it. In the renal system, bicarbonate is excreted through the kidneys. In the respiratory system, bicarbonate is exhaled in the form of carbon dioxide.

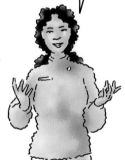

Measuring carbon dioxide is another way to evaluate pH balance. It can also help the physician evaluate overall renal function.

NONPROTEIN NITROGENOUS COMPOUNDS

In addition to measuring electrolytes, physicians also may measure three nonprotein **nitrogenous** compounds to help assess renal function. Nitrogenous means relating to, or containing, nitrogen.

When renal function is compromised, urea, creatinine, and uric acid can build up in the blood. However, other conditions also can affect the concentrations of these substances. For this reason, measuring the levels of nonprotein nitrogenous compounds in the blood isn't an absolute indicator of renal function. See the table on page 207 for more information about the following tests.

Blood Urea Nitrogen

Urea is a waste product that forms in the liver. It's the major end product of protein and amino acid metabolism. The body rids itself of urea by excreting it from the kidneys. Because both the liver and the kidneys process urea, measuring urea levels can tell the physician how the liver and kidneys are functioning.

Urea is usually measured by a chemistry test called BUN, which stands for blood urea nitrogen. (As you might expect, urea contains nitrogen.) The normal range for urea levels in the blood is 10 to 20 mg/dL.

Renal function and liver function aren't the only factors that affect BUN levels. Dietary intake of protein and a patient's level of hydration also affect the BUN level. In acute kidney conditions, the BUN increases before creatinine increases.

Creatinine

Creatinine is the waste product of **creatine.** Creatine is a chemical compound in the body that's used to store energy. When creatine is used, creatinine forms. While normal values vary somewhat among labs, the generally accepted normal range for creatinine in the blood is 0.8 to 1.4 mg/dL.

Measuring the creatinine present in a patient's blood is actually a better and more specific way to evaluate renal function than the BUN. Here's why. Only trace amounts of creatinine are reabsorbed by the renal system. So the urinary excretion of creatinine is about equal to the amount produced in the body. Urea, on the other hand, is reabsorbed to a certain extent, making it a less reliable indicator of renal function.

Uric Acid

Uric acid is a byproduct of protein metabolism in the blood. It's excreted by the kidneys. For men, the normal range is 3.5 to 7.2 mg/dL. For women, it's 2.6 to 6.0 mg/dL. Increased amounts of uric acid in the blood are more threatening than decreased amounts.

Hyperuricemia (uric acid levels above the normal range) can occur when a patient experiences renal failure. High uric acid levels are also found in patients undergoing chemotherapy for leukemias and other cancers.

Diets high in proteins (meat, legumes, and yeast) also can cause mild hyperuricemia. Such diets can aggravate a disease called **gout,** especially if they include food high in a group of amino acids called purines. All meats, fish, and poultry contain purines. But high amounts are found in organ meats like liver, kidney, or brain, as well as in seafood like scallops, shrimp, and anchovies.

Ask the Professional · GIVING MEDICAL ADVICE TO PATIENTS

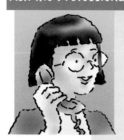

Q: *A patient who's been diagnosed with gout asked me if he should modify his diet. I told him that he should limit his alcohol intake and not eat too much meat because I know both of those things can aggravate gout. A coworker overheard me and told me that I'm not qualified to hand out this advice. I know my information is correct, so what did I do wrong?*

A: Your coworker is right. As a medical assistant, you should not give medical advice, even when you think you're correct. Giving any medical advice to patients without the physician telling you to do so falls outside your scope of practice.

What you should have done was ask the physician. Many patients with gout are prescribed a low-purine diet at first. Foods high in purine include organ meats such as hearts, livers, and kidneys, as well as sweetbreads, sardines, mackerel, herring, and anchovies.

Often, dietary changes along with medication can keep gout under control. But you must remember that a physician or registered dietician should offer such dietary teaching. Your information was correct, but it was incomplete. That makes it a disservice to the patient.

Patients with gout have a high uric acid buildup in their joints; the joints become inflamed and painful. Uric acid is usually not tested for in synovial fluid (joint fluid), but the fluid may be examined under a microscope for the presence of uric acid crystals.

Tests for Liver Function

The liver is the largest gland in the body and one of the most complex. Some of its major functions include:

- the production of **bile** (the bitter yellow-green secretion of the liver that's stored in the gallbladder)
- the metabolism of many compounds used by the body
- the processing of bilirubin
- detoxifying substances in the blood

To help evaluate liver function, these tests are commonly performed:

- bilirubin
- alkaline phosphatase (ALP)
- alanine aminotransferase (ALT)
- aspartate aminotransferase (AST)
- albumin

BILIRUBIN

Bilirubin is a substance that's produced as a byproduct of hemoglobin breakdown. If too much bilirubin settles into the skin and sclera (the fibrous tissue covering the eye), the patient appears amber, or jaundiced. That's because bilirubin is amber in color.

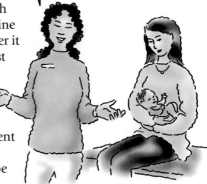

Bilirubin causes many newborns to appear jaundiced, or yellow, a few days after birth. Often, a newborn's liver isn't developed enough to remove bilirubin from the blood.

Bilirubin is frequently measured, along with liver enzymes present in the blood, to determine the health of the liver. The liver's ability to filter it from the blood is one of the first functions lost in many liver diseases. That's why elevated levels of bilirubin in a patient's blood or urine can be a sign of early liver disease.

Bilirubin can be broken down by fluorescent light or sunlight. Any specimen (blood or urine) that will be tested for bilirubin must be protected from exposure to light.

HOW THE BODY MAKES BILIRUBIN

Here's how the body makes and excretes bilirubin.

1. Red blood cells live about 120 days; the liver and spleen remove worn-out RBCs from circulation.
2. Part of the hemoglobin in the worn-out cells breaks down into bilirubin.
3. The bilirubin travels through the bloodstream to the liver, which passes it on to the gallbladder.
4. In the gallbladder, the bilirubin becomes part of a fluid called bile. It passes to the small intestine when bile is added to food being digested.

5. Bacteria in the intestinal tract convert the bilirubin into two forms—urobilin and urobilirubin. The urobilin is excreted in feces. Most of the urobilirubin is carried back to the liver in the blood.

A small amount of urobilirubin is filtered from the blood by the kidneys and excreted in urine. The rest is removed from the blood by the liver.

LIVER ENZYMES

An enzyme is a protein produced by living cells that speeds up chemical reactions. Three of the enzymes present in the liver are:

- alkaline phosphatase (ALP)
- alanine aminotransferase (ALT)
- aspartate aminotransferase (AST)

Alkaline Phosphatase

Let's look at each of these enzymes in a little more detail. For example, alkaline phosphatase (ALP) exists in the following places in the body:

- bones
- liver
- intestines
- kidneys
- placenta

The ALP circulating in the blood is mostly from the liver and bone. If a patient has a liver or bone disorder, serum ALP levels will rise. Normal ranges for ALP vary depending on the age of the patient.

High levels of ALP are considered normal during periods of bone growth. Examples of such times would be childhood growth spurts and during the third trimester of pregnancy.

Alanine Aminotransferase and Aspartate Aminotransferase

The enzymes alanine aminotransferase (ALT) and aspartate aminotransferase (AST) are present in many organs. Organ damage, such as damage to the heart or liver, can result in increased levels of ALT and AST in the blood. Some medications can also cause an increase in ALT or AST.

ALBUMIN

Albumin testing is also part of many liver profiles. Albumin is the smallest and most plentiful of the blood proteins. It binds and transports substances in the blood. Albumin also helps to maintain fluid balance in the body's tissues.

Decreased levels of albumin can be due to several factors:

- malnutrition and muscle-wasting diseases
- liver disease that makes the liver cells unable to produce albumin
- excessive loss in urine due to renal disease
- inflammation of the intestinal tract
- burns

Closer Look — TESTING FOR DRUG-RELATED LIVER DAMAGE

One of the liver's functions is detoxification. With most substances, the liver performs this function with little or no ill effects. Occasionally, drugs or the products of drug breakdown can have harmful effects on the liver.

The physician can detect this damage by measuring enzymes (AST, ALT, and alkaline phosphatase) released into the blood. The greater the damage to the liver, the higher the blood levels of these enzymes will be.

Small elevations in these enzymes may be acceptable if the drug is helping the patient. The dose may be adjusted or the drug stopped while the physician weighs its benefits against the risk of possible harm to the liver. The physician may look for another drug instead, in hopes of reducing or eliminating the harmful effects.

With certain drugs, the patient's enzyme levels must be monitored throughout the course of the treatment. Checking them once is not enough. That's because a drug may be tolerated for a period of time with no increase in enzymes. Then, suddenly, the cumulative effects of taking the drug will result in a sudden increase in enzyme levels.

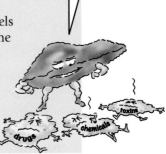

The liver helps protect the body by eliminating drugs, harmful chemicals, and biological toxins.

Tests for Thyroid Function

The thyroid gland regulates the body's metabolism by secreting two hormones—triiodothyronine and thyroxine. The thyroid gland itself is controlled by another hormone, called thyroid-stimulating hormone, or TSH. This hormone is produced in the anterior pituitary gland, located at the base of the brain.

When no disease is present and additional thyroid hormones are needed, the anterior pituitary gland secretes more TSH to stimulate the thyroid gland. When lesser amounts of the hormones are required, the anterior pituitary gland secretes less TSH. Less TSH causes the thyroid gland to reduce its production of the other hormones.

Many situations can cause an imbalance in this delicate **endocrine system.** The endocrine system is made up of hormones and the glands that secrete them. In the endocrine system, all secretions are internal, meaning into the bloodstream.

When the anterior pituitary gland malfunctions, it creates an oversecretion or an undersecretion of TSH. If the thyroid gland isn't working properly, it can't be stimulated no matter how much TSH is secreted. In cases such as these, TSH levels may be very high. In addition to TSH, the tests triiodothyronine (T3) and thyroxin (T4) are commonly ordered in the investigation of thyroid problems.

Tests for Cardiac Function

When a myocardial infarction occurs, the damaged heart muscle releases large quantities of certain enzymes into the bloodstream. A myocardial infarction, also known as a heart attack, is the death of cardiac muscle due to a lack of blood flow to the muscle. The two enzymes released are creatine kinase-MB and troponin.

CREATINE KINASE-MB

Creatine kinase (CK) is found in three places in the body:

- skeletal muscle
- myocardium (the middle layer of the walls of the heart)
- nervous tissue (in the brain)

CK has three **isoenzymes.** Isoenzymes are enzymes that are chemically different, but functionally the same. That means that although the isoenzymes each have their own chemical properties, they all perform the same job. The three isoenzymes of CK are called:

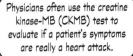

Physicians often use the creatine kinase-MB (CKMB) test to evaluate if a patient's symptoms are really a heart attack.

- MM (muscle enzyme)
- MB (heart enzyme)
- BB (brain enzyme)

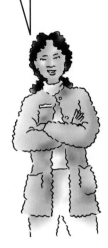

When a patient has chest pain, CKMB levels, along with total CK, are tested to determine whether the patient has had a heart attack. For two to eight hours after a myocardial infarction, CKMB levels rise and remain high for about 24 hours. They then return to normal if there is no new heart damage. CK levels also increase in crushing injuries, such as those received in car accidents.

Most of the normal levels of CK consist of the MM element. The MB level rises with myocardial infarction. A high total CK can indicate damage to either the heart or to other muscles, but a high CKMB suggests that the damage was to heart muscle.

TROPONIN

Troponin is a protein specific to heart muscle. It's a valuable tool in diagnosing acute myocardial infarction. Troponin levels in the blood begin to rise within four hours after myocardial damage has occurred. These levels may stay elevated for up to 14 days. Troponin levels are used to evaluate the extent of cardiac damage and to help the physician develop a prognosis for the patient.

Tests for Pancreatic Function

The pancreas is a gland that functions in both the endocrine system and the **exocrine system** and produces many secretions. In the exocrine system, secretions are outward onto the skin or into the body cavities. Exocrine glands include the salivary glands, sweat glands, and glands in the gastrointestinal tract.

Amylase and **lipase** are two exocrine system products of the pancreas. They are released as enzymes into the intestines to help digestion. Insulin and glucagon, two endocrine system products of the pancreas, are released into the bloodstream to regulate carbohydrate metabolism.

TESTING PANCREATIC ENZYMES

Amylase and lipase levels are tested to detect pancreatitis. Pancreatitis is an inflammation of the pancreas. When a patient has pancreatitis, the level of amylase in the blood increases quite a bit. The salivary glands also produce amylase, so when a patient has any of the inflammatory diseases of the salivary glands (such as mumps), the level of amylase rises as well.

Lipase levels also rise with pancreatitis. For a **differential diagnosis** of pancreatitis, both enzymes should be measured. A differential diagnosis is a systematic way of figuring out exactly what disease a patient has. Physicians weigh the probability of one disease against another based on test results.

PANCREATIC HORMONES AND CARBOHYDRATE METABOLISM

Sugar has several chemical forms. One of them is glucose. Glucose is a primary source of energy for the body. When the body metabolizes foods, nutrients including glucose are released into the bloodstream. Blood glucose levels must stay within narrow limits, however, or a person will experience negative physical effects. The pancreatic hormones insulin and glucagon help keep blood glucose levels within the appropriate range.

Insulin

Insulin brings the glucose into the body's cells. There, it's either used for energy or stored for future use. If enough energy is available for the cells to use, the extra glucose is stored as **glycogen** in the liver and muscles, or as fat. Glycogen is the stored form of glucose; it's made up of long chains of glucose.

Insulin is an important hormone. Cells starve if insulin isn't available or if they can't bring glucose in for energy. Also, by helping with glucose storage, insulin keeps blood glucose levels down. The result is that the body is able to maintain a stable normal range of glucose.

Glucagon

Glucagon is the hormone that stimulates the release of glycogen. Whenever blood glucose levels drop, the glucagon acts on the glycogen. It breaks it apart so that molecules of glucose are available for the cells to use. As a result, blood glucose levels rise again.

COMMON GLUCOSE TESTS

There are several tests a physician can order to determine how well the body's glucose metabolism system is working. These tests include:

- *Random blood glucose.* The specimen can be drawn at any time. The normal result is 60 to 126 mg/dL. Although this test isn't as useful as an FBS, it's a good screening tool.
- *Fasting blood sugar (FBS).* A blood glucose level is obtained following an 8- to 12-hour fast in which the patient ingests nothing but water.
- *Two-hour postprandial glucose (PP).* A blood sample is drawn two hours after a meal and the glucose level is measured.
- *Glucose tolerance test (GTT).* Blood glucose levels are checked at intervals after the patient takes a large dose of glucose.

Fasting Blood Sugar

The main purpose of determining a fasting glucose level is to detect either diabetes mellitus (usually just called *diabetes*) or

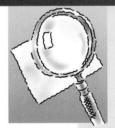

Closer Look GLUCOSE METERS

The glucose meter is a quick, accurate, easy, and relatively inexpensive way to measure a patient's blood glucose level in an office setting. Glucose meters are sold under many brand names. With proper instruction, patients can also use these devices to measure their own glucose levels at home. You'll read about instructing patients on how to use a glucose meter later in this chapter.

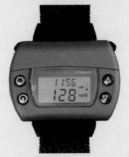
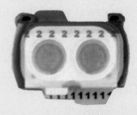

The Cygnus, Inc. GlucoWatch G2® Biographer is just one example of a small personal glucose meter. This glucose meter clips to the end of a person's finger and uses infrared light to determine the blood glucose level.

hypoglycemia (very low blood sugar). This test can be performed in the medical office or by the patient at home, using a glucose meter. For specific information on how to find an FBS level using a glucose meter, see the Hands On procedure on page 208.

The American Diabetes Association's cutoff point for normal fasting blood glucose levels is 100 mg/dL. A result of 100 to 125 mg/dL indicates a condition called *prediabetes*. This means the person has higher-than-normal glucose levels, but not high enough to diagnose diabetes. A diagnosis of diabetes requires a fasting blood glucose of 126 mg/dL or above. Studies show that many people with prediabetes develop diabetes within ten years.

A two-hour PP or a GTT is often performed to confirm a high FBS result. A GTT is also used to diagnose hypoglycemia. Hypoglycemia is characterized by FBS levels below 45 mg/dL. A number of symptoms are associated with very low blood glucose levels. These symptoms include:

- sweating
- weakness
- dizziness
- headache
- trembling
- lethargy

Two-Hour Postprandial Glucose

The purpose of the two-hour PP is to screen patients for diabetes and to monitor insulin therapy of diabetic patients. Before the test, the patient must first fast for 12 hours and then eat a high-carbohydrate meal. As a substitute for the meal, patients may drink a glucose solution instead. The standard glucose drink for this test contains 100 grams of glucose. The patient can eat exactly 300 grams of spaghetti, rice, baked potato, or 150 grams of white bread. This is equivalent to about 75 grams of sugar. Then, two hours later, a blood sample is drawn and the patient's glucose level is measured. Correct timing of the blood collection is extremely important in this test. "Good control" of diabetes is defined by a two-hour PP value of less than 140 mg/dL.

The physician may adjust the quantity of grams based on the patient's body weight.

Glucose Tolerance Test

The GTT is used to diagnose diabetes and hypoglycemia. The patient ingests a large dose of glucose. Then, blood glucose levels are checked at 30 minutes and 1, 2, and 3 hours after the glucose has been ingested. This checks how the body is metabolizing the glucose. The GTT follows a check of the fasting glucose. For the exact steps in performing a GTT, see the Hands On procedure on page 211.

As in a two-hour PP, the blood samples must be drawn at the exact times for the diagnosis to be valid. A serum or plasma specimen can be collected, depending on what the lab requires. It's also possible that urine specimens may be collected from the patient during the timed intervals.

The blood specimens should be centrifuged and separated as soon as possible to prevent the red blood cells from metabolizing the glucose. However, specimens that are collected in gray stopper tubes containing sodium fluoride are stable for up to three days even without centrifuging.

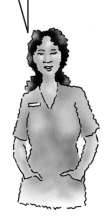

A low-carb diet of less than 150 grams of carbohydrates per day will produce an abnormal Glucose Tolerance Test result.

Hypoglycemia and the Glucose Tolerance Test. Hypoglycemia may also be diagnosed by the GTT, but the test may be extended by additional blood collections at four, five, and six hours after the glucose was ingested. You must watch your patient carefully. If she experiences any of the symptoms of hypoglycemia, you must draw a blood specimen even if it's not time for one yet.

Unfortunately, a glucose level that's lower than the normal range often does not correspond to the patient's symptoms. The patient's emotional state or level of anxiety, not low glucose levels, may cause the symptoms. Frequently, these same patients improve when their food intake is divided so that they eat many small meals rather than several large ones. This way, smaller glucose loads are introduced to the body.

Interpreting Glucose Tolerance Test Results. As a medical assistant, you won't interpret the results of the GTT. Many methods are used to interpret the values from a GTT. However, the National Diabetes Data Group and the World Health Organization proposed criteria that are endorsed by the American Diabetes Association. These criteria recommend a diagnosis of diabetes if the fasting glucose level is greater than 110 mg/dL and the two-hour measurement is equal to or above 155 mg/dL.

Diabetic Glucose Testing

As you know, blood glucose levels are used to monitor diabetic patients as well as to diagnose diabetes. The preferred test for monitoring patients already known to have diabetes is the hemoglobin A_1C test. The normal glycated hemoglobin (Hb A_1C) is less than 6.05 percent. The ideal glycated hemoglobin (Hb A_1C) for a known diabetic is less than seven percent.

The hemoglobin A_1C test measures the average amount of glucose that's been circulating in the patient's blood over a three-month period. In comparison, a venipuncture specimen or a finger stick measurement gives only the amount of glucose in the blood at the time of the test.

OBSTETRIC GLUCOSE TESTING

Some pregnant patients have increased glucose intolerance in their second and third trimesters. A pregnant patient's glucose level must be monitored because **gestational diabetes** can endanger the fetus. Gestational diabetes occurs during pregnancy when a woman's body is not metabolizing carbohydrates properly. Usually, this happens because the patient develops an insulin deficiency. This condition usually disappears after delivery.

The most common way to screen a pregnant patient for gestational diabetes is to have her drink a 50 g glucose load and then draw her blood one hour later. This test is usually performed during the second trimester. If the test result shows a blood glucose level over 155 mg/dL, a GTT is ordered to confirm a diagnosis of gestational diabetes.

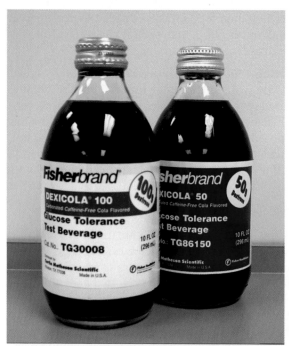

Most commercial glucose tolerance test beverages are either 50 g or 100 g. Patients sometimes find it easier to drink the test beverage if it is very cold.

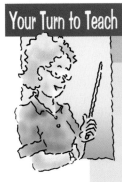

Your Turn to Teach

HELPING PATIENTS USE A GLUCOSE METER

Diabetic patients often have to monitor their own glucose levels. As a medical assistant, you can help them understand the procedure so they can perform it at home without difficulty. You should help the patient get familiar with her glucose meter. Instruct the patient to closely follow all the manufacturer's instructions. Also stress the following points with these patients.

- Make sure patients understand the need to test and document their glucose levels regularly. Help them understand why this is so important.

- Following the manufacturer's instructions, instruct patients how to maintain a quality control record for their meters. Demonstrate by using the control materials provided by the manufacturer. Remind patients to pay attention to the expiration date on the control materials.

- Explain the proper technique for getting a blood sample—for example, cleansing the area well before the finger stick and not milking the finger afterward.

- Caution patients not to self-regulate their glucose levels with insulin. Tell them to call the physician if glucose levels are abnormal.

- Make sure patients know the signs and symptoms of high and low glucose levels and the treatments for each.

The Hands On procedure on page 208 also can be used to guide patients in doing their own glucose meter tests.

> Most pharmacies and medical supply stores that sell glucose meters also teach patients how to use them.

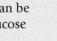

TESTS FOR LIPIDS AND LIPOPROTEINS

To assess the risk for heart disease, a physician orders tests to measure the amounts of the following substances present in a patient's blood:

- cholesterol
- **lipids** (free fatty acids)
- **lipoproteins** (substances made up of lipids and proteins)

MEDICAL WASTE DISPOSAL

As a medical assistant, you may be responsible for obtaining blood specimens for chemistry testing. It's extremely important that you dispose of all soiled or contaminated materials in the proper way. In the physician's office, there are three basic types of waste containers—the regular waste container, the sharps waste container, and the biohazard waste container. Follow these guidelines to dispose of medical waste properly.

Use the regular waste container for waste that's not biohazardous. Some examples include:

- paper
- plastic
- disposable tray wrappers
- packaging material
- unused gauze

Use the sharps waste container for sharp objects that could puncture or injure someone. Examples of sharps are:

- needles
- syringes
- lancets
- scalpels
- broken glass

Use the biohazard waste container for waste contaminated with blood or body fluids. Some examples of biohazardous waste include:

- soiled examination gloves
- cotton balls, applicators, or gauze that has been used on the body
- soiled dressings and bandages
- soiled examination table paper
- anything, including used glucose meter reagent strips, that has blood or body fluids on it

While these compounds have been associated with heart disease for a long time, they're also important building blocks of our bodies. They're part of every cell membrane and of the myelin sheath around the nerves. They also cushion and support organs. The key is that these compounds exist in the body in proper quantities.

Cholesterol

It seems as though cholesterol is only known for the problems it can cause. But actually, cholesterol performs important body functions. Here are just some of the ways that cholesterol is important.

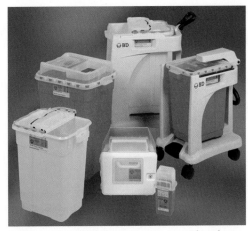

Here are several styles of sharps containers used for safety in the medical office.

- Cholesterol helps form bile acids that are produced in the liver and stored in the gallbladder. These bile acids are released into the intestine for the digestion of fats.
- Vitamin D is formed from cholesterol at the skin's surface during exposure to sunlight.
- Various hormones, such as cortisol, testosterone, and estrogen, are synthesized from cholesterol.

Only when cholesterol exceeds the levels necessary for cell maintenance and other body functions should it be considered a health hazard.

The American Heart Association recommends that the cholesterol level in the blood be less than 200 mg/dL. Anyone with a level above 200 mg/dL is considered to be at an increased risk for developing **atherosclerosis.** This condition involves the buildup of fatty

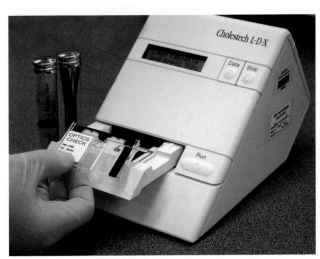

Analyzers such as this one can measure levels of cholesterol, triglycerides, low-density lipoprotein, and high-density lipoprotein in the blood.

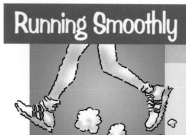

Running Smoothly

HELPING ENSURE ACCURATE LIPID MEASUREMENTS

How can you help get the most accurate test results for the patient and the physician?

Many factors can affect the results of a lipid profile. To a large extent, neither you nor the laboratory can control these factors. But there are some things you can do to help reduce factors that can affect the results.

- Make sure the patient has not performed vigorous physical activity in the 24 hours before testing. Lipids and lipoproteins should be measured only when the patient is in a steady metabolic state.

- Ask the patient to remain seated for at least five minutes before the blood is drawn.

- Verify that the patient has maintained his usual diet and weight for at least two weeks before the test.

- Fasting or nonfasting specimens can be used for total cholesterol testing. But a 12-hour fasting specimen is required for triglycerides and lipoproteins. Make sure you know which type of specimen you need.

- Total cholesterol, triglyceride, and HDL concentrations can be determined in either serum or plasma. Heparin is the preferred anticoagulant if plasma is to be used. Avoid EDTA.

- Multiple measurements within two months, at least one week apart, should be performed before a medical decision about further action is made.

plaque on the interior lining of arteries, causing the arteries to narrow and harden.

Low-Density Lipoprotein

Low-density lipoprotein (LDL) is a protein found in blood plasma that carries cholesterol from the liver to the walls of large and medium-sized arteries. Sometimes, the fatty plaque of atherosclerosis builds up in the arteries. This narrows and thickens the affected vessel and it becomes more rigid. Another result is reduced circulation to the organs and other areas normally supplied by these arteries.

Atherosclerosis is the major cause of coronary heart disease, angina pectoris (chest pain due to a lack of oxygen to the heart), myocardial infarction, and other cardiac illnesses. As you might expect, when LDL values are above the normal range, the risk of heart disease increases. Normal levels of LDL are less than 100 mg/dL. Levels above 129 mg/dL are considered borderline high, and any figure above 159 mg/dL can be dangerously high.

High-Density Lipoprotein

High-density lipoprotein (HDL) is the protein molecule that carries cholesterol from the walls of the arteries back to the liver. HDL is commonly referred to as the "good cholesterol." Usually, HDL levels are lower than those for LDL. In men, average HDL levels range from 40 to 50 mg/dL. For women, the average is 50 to 60 mg/dL.

Researchers have been investigating whether there's a way to increase HDL, because higher levels of HDL seem to lower the incidence of heart disease. Unlike LDL, that means the *lower* a patient's HDL level, the *greater* the patient's risk for heart disease. Therefore, with HDL, higher levels are better.

Closer Look   CALCULATING A PATIENT'S CARDIAC RISK

Using a simple calculation, you can give patients an estimation of their cardiac risk. Here's how. Divide the patient's total cholesterol figure by his HDL figure. A result of four indicates normal cardiac risk. A number less than four indicates a lower than normal cardiac risk, and a number more than four indicates an increased cardiac risk. The table on the next page shows the results for three fictional patients.

The table shows that patient B has the highest cardiac risk even though he has the lowest total cholesterol level. And patient C, with the highest total cholesterol, has the lowest risk. These results show the importance of HDL in maintaining good heart health.

Examples of Cardiac Risk

Patient	Total Cholesterol (mg/dL)	HDL (mg/dL)	Result	Cardiac Risk
A	180	45	4	Normal
B	150	25	6	Increased (less healthy)
C	210	70	3	Decreased (healthier)

Triglycerides

Triglycerides store energy. They're stored in adipose tissue (body tissue that stores fat) and muscle and released and metabolized between meals according to the body's energy demands. Adipose (fatty) tissue is almost completely made up of triglycerides.

Normal triglyceride levels vary according to a person's age and gender. However, in general, the level should be less than 150 mg/dL. Research has identified high triglyceride levels (200 mg/dL or more) as a risk factor in heart disease.

Many people with high triglycerides can bring down their levels through weight loss, regular exercise, and diet. They should limit their intake of carbohydrates to not more than 50 percent of their total calories, This is because carbohydrates raise triglycerides in some people and lower HDL cholesterol.

Legal Brief   TEST RESULTS AND PATIENT PRIVACY

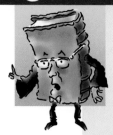

As a medical assistant, you'll have access to sensitive test results that have great importance to a patient's state of health. For example, in this chapter, you read about tests that show if a patient has diabetes and others that can show if a patient is at high risk for a heart attack or a stroke.

You must remember that a patient's health status is her own personal information. You have a responsibility to keep the results of these tests, as well as *all* test results and other medical information, from unauthorized persons. Only the physician and the patient are entitled to test results. The only exception is when laws require reporting certain test results to protect public health and safety. However, deciding when to do this won't be your responsibility.

Common Chemistry Panel Tests

Test	Body Function	Normal Value	Causes of Increase	Causes of Decrease
BUN	Metabolic byproduct	10–20 mg/dL	Kidney disease, kidney obstruction, dehydration	Liver failure, malnutrition
Calcium	Structural element for bones, teeth, muscles	8.5–10.5 mg/dL	Hyperparathyroidism, hyperthyroidism, Addison's disease, bone cancer, multiple myeloma, other malignancies	Hypoparathyroidism, renal failure
Chloride	Acid-base balance, component of stomach acid	96–110 mEq/L	Dehydration, Cushing's syndrome, hyperventilation	Severe vomiting, severe diarrhea, severe burn, pyloric obstruction, heat exhaustion
Cholesterol	Building block for cell membranes, steroid hormones, bile acids	120–200 mg/dL	Atherosclerosis, heart disease, certain liver diseases with obstruction, hypothyroidism	Liver disease, hyperthyroidism, malabsorption syndrome
Creatinine	Metabolic byproduct	0.8–1.4 mg/dL	Kidney disease, muscle disease	Muscular dystrophy
Glucose	Energy source	60–100 mg/dL	Diabetes mellitus, Cushing's syndrome, liver disease	Excessive insulin, Addison's disease, bacterial sepsis, hypothyroidism
Phosphorus	Used in bone, endocrine processes	2.5–4.5 mg/dL	Renal disease, hypoparathyroidism, hypocalcemia, Addison's disease	Hyperparathyroidism, bone disease
Potassium	Acid-base balance	3.5–5.0 mEq/L	Kidney disease, cell damage, Addison's disease	Diarrhea, starvation, severe vomiting, severe burn, some liver diseases
Sodium	Fluid balance	135–145 mEq/L	Dehydration, Cushing's syndrome, diabetes insipidus	Severe burns, diarrhea, vomiting, Addison's disease
Triglycerides	Energy source; lipid deposits for stored energy, organ support	Men: 40–160 mg/dL Women: 35–135 mg/dL	Atherosclerosis, liver disease, poorly controlled diabetes, pancreatitis	Malnutrition
Uric acid	Metabolic byproduct	Men: 3.5–7.2 mg/dL Women: 2.6–6.0 mg/dL	Renal failure, gout, leukemia, eclampsia	Drug therapy to lower uric acid levels

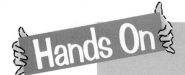

DETERMINING BLOOD GLUCOSE

The purpose of the blood glucose test is to measure the level of glucose in the blood for diagnosis and treatment of hypoglycemia and hyperglycemia. Follow these steps for using a glucose meter to determine blood glucose correctly:

1. Gather your equipment and supplies: a glucose meter of the physician's choice, glucose reagent strips, a lancet, an alcohol pad, sterile gauze, a paper towel, an adhesive bandage, and gloves.

2. Wash your hands and put on your gloves before you remove the reagent strip from the container.

3. Turn on the glucose meter and make sure that it's calibrated correctly. Otherwise, the test results may be inaccurate.

4. Remove one reagent strip, lay it on the paper towel, and recap the container. The strip is ready for testing and the paper towel serves as a disposable work surface. It will also absorb any excess blood.

5. Greet and identify the patient. Explain the procedure, and ask for and answer any questions the patient might have. Ask the patient when she last ate and document this in her chart.

6. Cleanse the puncture site (finger) with alcohol.

7. Perform a capillary puncture, following the steps outlined in Chapter 2. Wipe away the first drop of blood.

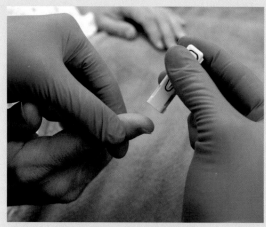

Pierce the patient's finger with a lancet.

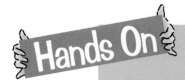

DETERMINING BLOOD GLUCOSE (continued)

6-1

8. Turn the patient's hand palm down and gently squeeze the finger so that a large drop of blood forms. You must squeeze gently to avoid diluting the sample with tissue fluid.

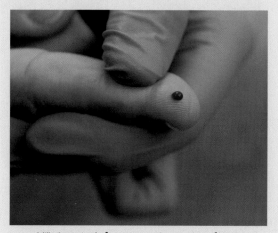

Milk the patient's finger to get a hanging drop of blood.

9. Bring the reagent strip up to the finger and touch the strip to the blood. Make sure you don't touch the finger. Then insert the reagent strip into the glucose meter.

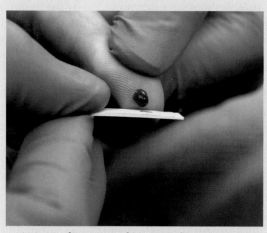

Apply drop of blood hanging from patient's finger to test strip.

(continued)

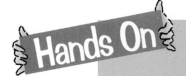

**DETERMINING BLOOD
GLUCOSE** (*continued*)

6-1

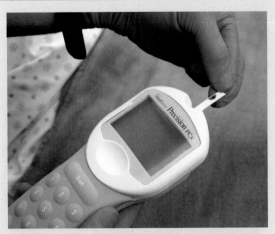

Place strip into meter.

10. Apply pressure to the puncture wound with gauze. While you are doing this, the meter will incubate the strip and measure the reaction.

11. The instrument reads the reaction strip and displays the result on the screen in milligrams per deciliter (mg/dL). If the glucose level is higher or lower than expected, review the troubleshooting guide provided by the manufacturer. Controls are available in the low, normal, and high range to ensure that the glucose meter is functioning properly. These controls should be run daily according to the manufacturer's instructions.

12. Apply a small adhesive bandage to the patient's fingertip.

13. Care for and dispose of your equipment and supplies. Clean your work area. Then you can remove your gloves and wash your hands.

Note: These are generic instructions for using a glucose meter. Use the package insert to get specific instructions for the meter you are using.

Charting Example:
02/12/2007 10:00 A.M. Capillary puncture right middle finger. Glucose tested with Glucometer. Results: 60 mg/dL. Dr. Peters notified. _____ M. Miller, CMA

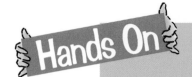

GLUCOSE TOLERANCE TESTING

6-2

The purpose of the glucose tolerance test (GTT) is to measure the body's ability to metabolize a premeasured quantity of glucose over a specified time. Follow these steps to accurately perform a glucose tolerance test:

1. Gather the following equipment and supplies: calibrated amount of glucose solution per physician's order, glucose meter equipment, phlebotomy equipment, glucose test strips, alcohol wipes, a stopwatch, and gloves. The stopwatch is particularly important because the timing of the blood collections has a direct effect on test results.

2. Greet and identify the patient. Explain the procedure, and ask for and answer any questions the patient might have. Ask the patient when he last ate and document this in his chart.

3. Wash your hands and put on your gloves.

4. Obtain a fasting glucose (FBS) specimen from the patient by venipuncture or capillary puncture as explained in Chapter 2.
   - It's recommended that a lab test the fasting blood sample before the patient ingests the glucose drink.
   - If the FBS exceeds 140 mg/dL, don't perform the test. Instead, inform the physician.
   - Giving more glucose to a patient whose blood glucose level is too high could seriously harm the patient.

5. Give the glucose drink to the patient and ask the patient to drink it all within five minutes. The body starts to metabolize the glucose right away, so the patient must drink rapidly.

6. Note the time the patient finishes the drink; this is the official start of the test. Keep the following things in mind during the test:
   - The patient should remain mostly inactive during this procedure because exercise alters the glucose levels by increasing the body's demand for energy.
   - The patient should not smoke during the test because smoking can artificially increase the glucose level.
   - The patient may drink water, but only water.
   - If the patient has any severe symptoms (for example, headache, dizziness, vomiting), obtain a blood specimen at that time. Then end the test and inform the physician. These symptoms could indicate intolerably high or low glucose levels.

(continued)

Hands On

7. Obtain another blood specimen exactly 30 minutes after the patient finishes the glucose drink. Label the specimen with the patient's name and time of collection. Follow the precautions listed in step 6 for the remainder of the test. The physician may want urine glucose tests done with each blood sample taken. Ask the patient to submit a urine sample after you take the blood sample. Never attempt to get the urine sample before the blood sample as it might cause you to miss the time for the blood sample. If the patient doesn't provide a urine sample, don't worry about it. Submit an empty urine cup in place or an actual urine sample and label "patient could not provide urine sample at _____ [time]." Note: It is absolutely vital to the accuracy of the test that you are precise with the timing of the blood collections. Make all proper notations so the results can be accurately interpreted.

8. Exactly one hour after the glucose drink, repeat step 7.

9. Exactly two hours after the glucose drink, repeat step 7.

10. Exactly three hours after the glucose drink, repeat step 7. Unless a test longer that three hours has been ordered, the test is now complete. Otherwise, continue with the test for the specified period of time. Sometimes, the test can be up to six hours to detect hypoglycemia.

11. If the specimens are going to be tested by an outside laboratory, package them carefully and arrange for transportation.

12. Care for and dispose of your equipment and supplies. Clean your work area. Then you can remove your gloves and wash your hands.

Charting Example:
12/08/2007 10:30 A.M. 08:00 GTT test
08:00 FBS: 100 mg/dL glucose
08:10 Glucose drink to pt.
08:15 Glucose drink finished
08:45 Glucose 125 mg/dL
09:15 Glucose 132 mg/dL
10:15 Glucose 120 mg/dL
11:15 Glucose 110 mg/dL
Pt. tolerated procedure well, discharged by Dr. Lynch.
_____ B. Smith, RMA

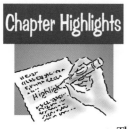

Chapter Highlights

- Blood chemistry tests measure important substances in serum, plasma, whole blood, and other body fluids.

- There are two main purposes for performing chemistry tests: (1) to evaluate organ function, and (2) to have a more complete understanding of a patient's overall health. Medical assistants should know what abnormal test results may mean.

- The current trend in clinical chemistry is to refer testing to reference laboratories where large automated analyzers are used. These automated analyzers can conduct tests at a lower cost than smaller labs. But no matter where tests are performed, the results are only as good as the specimen submitted for testing.

- Clinical chemistry tests can help evaluate the following: renal/kidney function, liver function, thyroid function, cardiac function and pancreatic function. Chemistry tests also measure the levels of lipids and lipoproteins as an indicator of the risks of heart disease.

- To evaluate renal/kidney function, tests measure electrolytes and nonprotein nitrogenous compounds in the blood.

- To assess liver function, these tests are commonly performed: bilirubin, serum albumin, alkaline phosphatase (ALP), alanine aminotransferase (ALT), aspartate aminotransferase (AST).

- The TSH (thyroid-stimulating hormone) test is the most common test ordered to check thyroid function.

- Myocardial infarction is evaluated by testing the enzymes creatine kinase-MB (CKMB) and troponin.

- Assessing pancreatic function includes testing for pancreatic enzymes such as amylase and lipase, as well as performing glucose tests of varying types.

- The risk of heart disease can be evaluated using the following tests as risk indicators: cholesterol, low-density lipoprotein (LDL), high-density lipoprotein (HDL), and triglycerides.

- A medical assistant must have a basic understanding of all aspects of the tests performed in the physician office lab, as well as a broad knowledge of tests sent out to larger labs for analysis. This knowledge must include the basic principles of the test, the proper sampling procedures, and the specific handling requirements for the specimen.

Chapter 7

MICROBIOLOGY

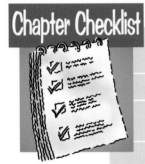

Chapter Checklist

- Describe how cultures are used in medical microbiology and explain what media and colonies are

- Name and describe the different types of bacteria

- Identify the main types of fungi that may be found in the human body

- Identify different types of viruses

- Identify the two main types of metazoa and give at least one example of each

- Summarize the medical assistant's responsibilities in microbiological testing

- List the most common microbiological specimens collected in the physician's office lab

- Collect a specimen for throat culture

- Collect a sputum specimen

- Collect a stool specimen

- Test a stool specimen for occult blood

- Explain how to transport a specimen

- State the difference between primary cultures, secondary cultures, and pure cultures

- Name at least three kinds of media used in cultures

- Explain how to care for media plates

- Summarize the ways of inoculating media

- Inoculate a culture using dilution streaking

- Inoculate for drug sensitivity testing using "even lawn" streaking

- Inoculate for quantitative culturing or urine colony count using "even lawn" streaking

- Describe how microscopic examination is used in medical microbiology

- Prepare a wet mount slide

- Prepare a dry smear

- State the purpose of Gram staining and summarize the process

- Gram stain a smear slide

You already know that the prefix *micro-* means "very small." So, it won't surprise you to find out that microbiology is the study of very small life. This small life includes bacteria, viruses, fungi, and parasites. For the most part, these microorganisms, or *microbes,* are so small that you can't see them without a microscope. But even though they're tiny, some microbes can still cause big health problems. Microorganisms that can cause disease are called **pathogens.**

Many microbes that don't cause disease, called **normal flora,** live in and on the human body without causing any problems. Some are even helpful to us. Many types of normal flora and pathogens thrive at temperatures between 96 degrees and 101 degrees F and in a fairly neutral environment. The human body typically offers these conditions.

As a medical assistant, you need to understand microbes and know the conditions in which they could become a problem for patients. Your understanding of microbiology will also help protect patients, your coworkers, and you from **nosocomial infections** (infections people can get from being in a medical setting).

Microbiological Testing

Medical microbiology involves testing to find out what kinds of microbes are living in a sample. This is often done by growing cultures from patients' specimens. A **culture** is colonies of bacteria grown under controlled conditions in a container in a

PREVENTING NOSOCOMIAL INFECTIONS

A physician's office often will be full of sick people. The lab that tests the office's specimens may be working with many types of pathogens. Health care professionals must take steps to protect themselves and others from infection. There are some common ways infections are spread in a medical setting.

- *Person to person.* This includes direct contact with patients who are ill as well as contact among coworkers.

- *Contaminated medical equipment.* Dirty instruments and needles fall into this category, along with other items such as medical laundry.

- *Bacteria in the environment.* This includes airborne transmission of microorganisms.

- *Failure to follow established procedures to avoid spreading microbes.* Some research indicates that nosocomial infections often result from a health care worker disregarding established procedures for infection control.

Here are steps you can take to protect yourself, coworkers, and patients from these infections.

- *Hand washing.* This is the single most important way to prevent nosocomial infections. Some research says that health care workers often think they're washing their hands more than they actually are. It also suggests that many workers aren't washing their hands long enough when they do wash them.

- *Gloves.* Gloves aren't a replacement for hand washing. They provide an extra layer of protection for you and the patient. Make sure you wear gloves whenever you'll be in contact with any body fluids. Also wear gloves when performing any kind of testing. When you remove contaminated gloves, be sure to follow the correct procedure and then wash your hands after your gloves have been removed.

- *Decontamination procedures.* You can reduce the risk of infection by strictly following procedures for cleaning, sanitizing, disinfecting, and sterilizing medical equipment. Plus, as you know, never try to reuse or clean single-use disposable items.

PREVENTING NOSOCOMIAL INFECTIONS (*continued*)

- *Single-use disposable equipment.* Whenever possible, use single-use disposable equipment and supplies. Make sure you dispose of medical waste properly.
- *Personal responsibility.* Take personal responsibility for your own safety and protection at work. Recognize that preventing the spread of microbes requires constant thought and attention.

lab. A **colony** is a group of identical bacteria that grow in a culture from one "parent" bacteria.

The purpose of growing a culture is to diagnose and treat a disease based on the kinds of bacteria present in the specimen. Cultures are grown in culture media with the help of an incubator. **Media** is special material in a container that helps bacteria present in the specimen to grow.

Specimens may be collected from different parts of the body. Here are some of the more common places:

- wounds
- throat
- vagina
- urethra
- skin

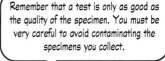

Remember that a test is only as good as the quality of the specimen. You must be very careful to avoid contaminating the specimens you collect.

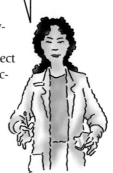

Specimens also may be drawn from the body, as in drawing blood, or excreted as sputum, stool, or urine.

As a medical assistant, it will often be your job to collect specimens or to assist the physician with specimen collection. You may collect specimens from wounds or from the throat, but the physician will usually collect specimens from the eye, ear, rectum, or reproductive organs. No matter how or where the specimens are collected, you must practice aseptic (sterile) technique so the specimen will provide accurate test results.

BACTERIA

Bacteria are one-celled simple organisms. Each type has its own characteristics. However, they all need four basic things to survive:

- nutrients
- warmth
- moisture
- gaseous composition of
  atmosphere
  — oxygen (for aerobic bacteria)
  — lack of oxygen (for anaerobic
     bacteria)
  — five to ten percent CO_2
     (for capnophilic bacteria)

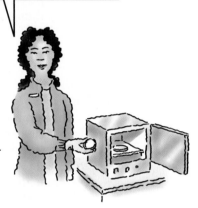

Using culture media and the incubator, you can grow cultures from patient specimens by simulating the four elements bacteria need to survive. Bacteria reproduce about every 20 minutes under the right conditions.

The human body provides all four requirements. Bacteria also can be created in the microbiology lab with the use of culture media and an incubator.

Bacteria can be identified by their own individual shapes, or morphology; chemical tests; and other ways, such as motility tests. There are several groups of bacteria, including the spore-forming bacteria that are very important in medical microbiology. On page 219, you can see high-power photos, taken through a microscope, of several types of these bacteria.

BACTERIOLOGY

Bacteriology is the science and study of bacteria. Organisms are named with both a genus and species name. The genus is always spelled with a capital letter, and the species begins with a lowercase letter (for example, *Staphylococcus aureus*). In print, the bacteria's name is italic or underlined. The name helps describe the characteristics of the bacterium (the singular form of the word *bacteria*) or the name or place connected with its discovery.

Cocci

The group of spherical bacteria—called **cocci**—cause many diseases. For example, species of **streptococci** (one genus of bacteria) may cause the following conditions:

- sore throat
- scarlet fever
- rheumatic fever

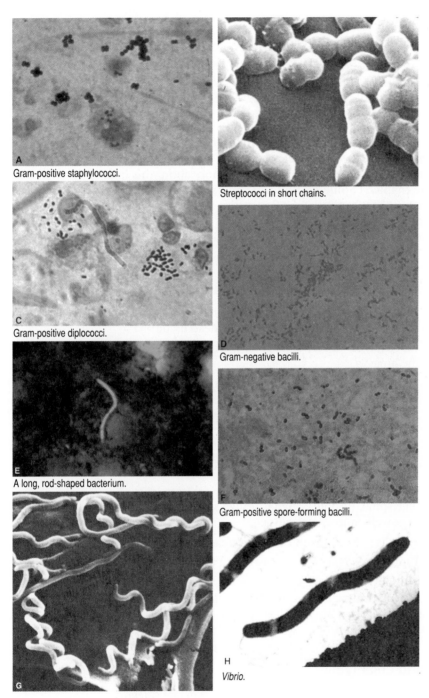

A
Gram-positive staphylococci.

Streptococci in short chains.

C
Gram-positive diplococci.

D
Gram-negative bacilli.

E
A long, rod-shaped bacterium.

F
Gram-positive spore-forming bacilli.

H
Vibrio.

G
The spirochete *Treponema pallidum* responsible for syphilis.

These photos show what different forms of bacteria look like under a microscope.

- many pneumonias
- a variety of skin infections

Certain species of **staphylococci** (another genus of bacteria) can be found on all surfaces of the skin and on many mucous membranes. Some of these bacteria also can cause skin infections.

Bacilli

Rod-shaped bacteria—called **bacilli**—usually need oxygen to live. This means they're **aerobic**. They also may be gram-positive or gram-negative. (You'll read more about this later in the chapter.) Some bacilli form **spores**. Spores are a form of bacteria that can resist the destructive forces of heat, drying, or chemicals.

Bacilli can cause many diseases, including:

- tetanus—a sometimes fatal infectious disease of the central nervous system
- botulism—a very serious form of food poisoning
- gas gangrene—a severe form of gangrene (death of living tissue) where gas is produced in the dead tissue
- tuberculosis—a very contagious infection usually found in the lungs
- pertussis—whooping cough, an infection of the respiratory system
- salmonellosis—another type of food poisoning
- certain pneumonias—respiratory infections
- otitis media—an infection in the middle ear

Spirochetes and Vibrios

The long, spiral, flexible bacteria—called **spirochetes**—cause disease as well. Spirochetes cause:

- syphilis (a sexually transmitted disease)
- Lyme disease (an illness caused by a tick bite)

Some spirochetes have **flagella,** or whiplike extensions that aid their movement. If the spiral bacteria are rigid (inflexible) rather than flexible, they're called spirilla.

The comma-shaped bacteria—called vibrios—are very motile. This means they move very well on their own too.

Rickettsias and Chlamydiae

Certain forms of bacteria fit into their own separate category. These forms are **rickettsias** and **chlamydiae.** They both share some common characteristics.

Closer Look BACTERIAL SPORES

Spores are extremely hardy forms of bacteria that are tough to kill. Some microbes can produce spores to protect themselves from destruction. Here's how it happens.

1. The bacterium, usually a bacillus (the singular form of the word *bacilli*), forms a capsule around itself.

2. Then it enters a resting state that keeps it from being destroyed through most attempts by asepsis to kill it.

3. Once the right conditions are again present, the bacterium picks up where it left off in its life cycle. It leaves its resting state and becomes active again.

Examples of bacteria that produce spores include:

- *Clostridium botulinum*—a bacteria that causes food poisoning
- *Clostridium tetani*—a bacteria that causes tetanus
- *Clostridium perfringens*—a bacteria that causes gas gangrene
- *Bacillus anthracis*—a bacteria that causes anthrax

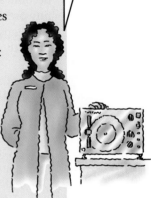

Bacterial spores can be destroyed using an autoclave set at just the right heat, steam, pressure, and time.

- They're smaller than bacteria but larger than viruses.
- They must have a living host to reproduce and survive. They're known as **obligate** intracellular parasites because they can't survive unless they're attached to a living host organism.

Rickettsias cause Rocky Mountain spotted fever, typhus, Q fever, trench fever, and others. The rickettsias are carried by a particular kind of tick, louse, or mite. Chlamydiae cause trachoma (an eye disease) and lymphogranuloma venereum (a sexually transmitted disease).

FUNGI

Like bacteria, fungi are small organisms that can produce disease given the right set of conditions. Also like bacteria, some fungi can be contagious as well as infectious. But fungi are more like plants, while bacteria are more like one-celled animals.

Many types of fungi can be seen with the naked eye, but some can only be seen under a microscope. **Mycology** is the science and study of fungi. Diseases caused by fungus are called mycotic infections, or mycoses.

In the human body, fungi can appear in the form of molds or yeasts. Tinea pedis (athlete's foot), tinea corporis (ringworm of the body), tinea capitis (ringworm of the scalp), and tinea unguium (nail fungus) are among the more common conditions caused by molds. Yeasts like candidiasis cause thrush (skin and mouth), vaginitis, and endocarditis. Candidiasis can be spread by contact. Fungi are **opportunistic,** which means they become able to cause disease when the opportunity presents itself. For example, fungi can cause problems when the host's normal flora can't offset the growth of the fungi.

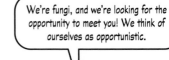

We're fungi, and we're looking for the opportunity to meet you! We think of ourselves as opportunistic.

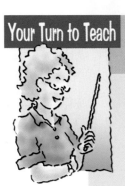

Your Turn to Teach

HELPING PATIENTS AVOID ATHLETE'S FOOT

One common fungal infection is tinea pedis, which is also known as athlete's foot. In spite of this name, patients don't have to be active in sports or even exercise to have this condition. You can help your patients avoid this irritating fungus by giving them the following guidelines.

- After a shower or a swim, dry your feet very thoroughly. Pay particular attention to drying between your toes.
- Wear water shoes or nonskid sandals anytime you're in a public shower or locker room. Don't walk around in your bare feet.
- Don't share shoes, slippers, sandals, or any other kind of footwear with anyone else.
- Use an antifungal powder between your toes. Sprinkle the powder in your shoes, too.
- Make sure your shoes can "breathe." Avoid plastic or vinyl shoes with no air circulation.
- Consider changing your socks once during the day to keep your feet drier. You should also alternate pairs of shoes. Wearing a pair only every other day gives shoes a chance to dry completely.

VIRUSES

Viruses are the smallest microorganisms, but they can be a lot of trouble for a patient. Viruses cause influenza, infectious hepatitis, rabies, polio, and AIDS. **Virology** is the study of viruses. These microbes are so tiny that they can't even be seen with the usual bright-field microscope found in many medical offices. They must be viewed under an electron microscope.

Like rickettsias and chlamydiae, viruses are obligate intracellular parasites. This means that they need a living host to survive and reproduce. However, unlike bacteria, antibiotics can't kill viruses. This makes most viruses difficult to treat. Scientists are developing antiviral therapies (drugs to slow or stop the growth of viruses) for many of the viruses. Researchers also continue to work on cures for viral diseases such as AIDS and herpes.

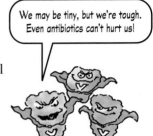

We may be tiny, but we're tough. Even antibiotics can't hurt us!

PROTOZOA AND METAZOA

Protozoa are the single-celled parasitic animals that may be diagnosed in the **parasitology** laboratory. Parasitology is the study of parasites and parasitism (a relationship in which one organism is dependent on another).

Here are some common protozoa and the conditions they cause:

- entamoeba—diarrhea, dysentery, and liver and lung disorders
- giardia—giardiasis, diarrhea, and malabsorption of nutrients
- trichomonas—trichomoniasis, vaginitis, and urinary tract infections
- plasmodium—malaria
- toxoplasma—toxoplasmosis and fetal abnormalities

Metazoa are also animal. However, they're multicellular rather than single-celled organisms like protozoa. Metazoa are of two types:

- helminths (parasitic worms)
- arthropods (animals with a hard external skeleton, segmented body, and jointed, paired legs)

The family of helminths includes roundworms (called nematodes), tapeworms (called cestodes), and flukes (called trematodes). They can survive almost anywhere in the human body. Some types can move through the body until they find a place to settle.

Flatworms

Trematodes and cestodes are both types of flatworms. They can cause these conditions:

- *Schistosomiasis.* Flukes (small, leaf-shaped flatworms) in contaminated water penetrate the skin and get into the bloodstream, bladder, and intestines.

- *Liver fluke infestation.* Flukes that live on plants or in fish in contaminated water enter the human body through the digestive tract. They migrate through the intestinal wall and settle in the bile ducts of the liver.

- *Beef or pork tapeworm infestation.* Humans can become infected by tapeworms when eating uncooked infected beef or pork. The parasite is separated from the meat during digestion in the stomach. It then moves into the small intestine where it attaches to the intestine's walls and develops into an adult tapeworm. An adult tapeworm can grow as long as 50 feet.

Roundworms

The nematodes also can infect humans. Here are some of the conditions they can cause.

- roundworm infestation (worms hatching and living in the intestines)
- gastrointestinal blockage
- bronchial damage
- pinworm infestation (worms filling the intestines and rectum)
- trichinosis (disease caused by eating undercooked pork or other wild game)

Arthropods

Arthropods are the better-known group of metazoa. They include mites, lice, ticks, fleas, bees, spiders, wasps, mosquitoes, and scorpions. All arthropods can cause injury with their bites or stings. Several also can transmit disease by biting or stinging.

Microbiology and You

Two main procedures are used to identify what possibly harmful bacteria may exist on or in a patient's body. These procedures are:

- *Culturing.* This means growing colonies of the bacteria present in a specimen in a carefully controlled environment in the lab.

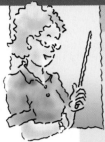

EDUCATING PATIENTS ABOUT LYME DISEASE

The deer tick is an arthropod that can transmit *Borrelia burgdorferi*, the spirochete that causes Lyme disease. The bacteria enters the human body when an infected tick bites a person. The bite results in symptoms that include:

- a bull's-eye shaped rash
- headache, fever, and chills
- fatigue and general body aches
- if left untreated, severe muscle, joint, heart, and nervous system problems

Teach patients to protect themselves from Lyme disease by giving them these guidelines.

- Try to avoid places where ticks live (for example, grassy, wooded, and bushy areas), especially in May–July when they are most active.

- Wear insect repellant, shoes, long socks, long pants, and long sleeves in outdoor areas to keep ticks off your skin. Light-colored clothing will make any ticks on it easier to see.

- Check your clothes each time you come inside after working or playing outdoors. Wash this clothing in hot water with strong soap.

- Perform daily checks for ticks after being outdoors. Include scalp and hair, groin, and armpits as well. Remove any ticks you find using fine-tipped tweezers. If a tick is attached to your skin for less than 24 hours, your chances of getting Lyme disease are small.

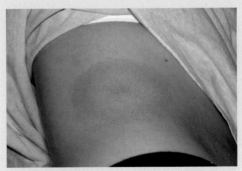

The appearance of a bull's-eye rash is associated with Lyme disease.

- *Microscopic examination.* This involves looking at the specimen through a microscope to identify any bacteria present in it.

As a medical assistant, you may be involved with both procedures in your medical office or lab. If you are, your responsibilities may be both administrative and clinical. Each medical setting is different. So you may perform tasks that medical assistants in other settings do not.

Your administrative duties may include:

- routing specimens
- handling and filing reports
- keeping patients safe
- educating patients
- billing and insurance filing

Your clinical duties may include:

- collecting and processing specimens
- assisting the physician and patient, as needed
- maintaining standard precautions and safety
- cleaning after testing is complete

COLLECTING SPECIMENS

As you know from your study of earlier chapters, physicians often obtain specimens from a patient's body to help them determine the state of the patient's health. Most lab tests are performed on specimens that are easy to collect. The most commonly tested specimens include:

- blood
- urine
- sputum
- feces
- wound drainage
- mucus from the throat and other parts of the body

Testing these substances can reveal much about a patient's condition. Here are just three of many examples.

- A throat culture can detect strep throat.
- A urine culture can show if there's an infection within the urinary system.

- A blood culture can detect infections in the circulatory system.

In Chapter 2, you learned how to collect blood specimens and in Chapter 5, you learned about the collection of urine specimens. This chapter includes information about how to collect other types of specimens, as well as instructions on how to conduct various microbiology tests.

To make sure these tests are accurate, you must collect specimens in the correct manner. You also must handle them according to accepted medical standards. Refer back to page 65 in Chapter 2 for a complete list of guidelines for collecting and handling specimens.

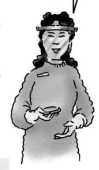

When collecting specimens, always follow proper procedure and avoid the temptation to take shortcuts.

COLLECTION METHODS

Most specimens for microbiological testing are obtained in one of four ways.

- *With a swab.* This is a stick topped with cotton or an absorbent manmade fiber. Swabs are used to take samples from the throat, vagina, urethra, skin, and wounds.

- *By venipuncture.* A syringe or butterfly needle is used to draw blood that's then deposited into special bottles so the blood can be cultured in the lab.

- *By centesis (surgical puncture).* This procedure will be performed by the physician. Specimens typically collected this way include spinal fluid and pleural fluid (fluid from lung membranes).

- *By collecting body excretions.* Examples include urine, sputum, and feces or stool. Patients usually collect these specimens on their own. It's important that they follow the proper collection technique.

Throat Cultures

The physician may order a throat culture to identify the presence of infectious microbes. A sterile swab gently sweeps the patient's throat to obtain the specimen. You also must use a tongue depressor for this procedure to avoid culturing mouth or cheek microbes that are normal flora. The Hands On procedure on page 244 provides the detailed procedure for obtaining a specimen for a throat culture.

Once the specimen is collected, it can be processed in two ways:

- in the office
- by sending it to an outside lab for analysis

If you send the swab to a lab, you must first place it in the correct culture medium. Then label the culture and put it in a biohazard bag. Be sure to include the proper paperwork requesting the test the physician has ordered. You'll read more about preparing specimens for testing by an outside lab a little later in this chapter.

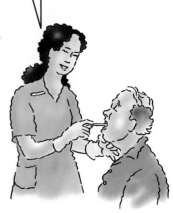

Throat cultures are useful when a patient has tonsillitis or a sore throat. The results of the throat culture help identify what's causing the problem.

Collecting Sputum

Sputum is mucus from a patient's lungs. It's often tested when diagnosing respiratory diseases such as pneumonia and tuberculosis. The specimen is collected by deep coughing. It's important that the specimen be a sample of lung secretions and not secretions from the mouth. For this reason, the patient should be instructed to avoid spitting saliva into the container.

It's best to obtain sputum specimens in the morning when the greatest volume is usually present in the lungs. If a patient's mucus is thick and difficult to cough up, a cool-mist humidifier might be ordered for him or her to use at home, to help loosen thick secretions.

You may be responsible for explaining sputum collection procedure to the patient. The Hands On procedure on page 245 provides step-by-step guidance on the proper method of collecting a sputum specimen.

Stool Specimens

Many physicians order a stool specimen as part of the routine physical exam of an adult patient. Appointments to collect stool specimens should be scheduled early in the morning. Most people move their bowels soon after getting up. Delaying the appointment may cause the patient discomfort or might result in loss of the specimen. In many cases, the patient may collect the sample at home. No matter where it's collected, it's important that the patient follow the proper procedure. You can use the Hands On procedure on page 246 as a guide for instructing patients about this.

Some stool specimens are collected and transported in special containers. It'll be your responsibility to make sure proper proce-

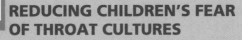 **REDUCING CHILDREN'S FEAR OF THROAT CULTURES**

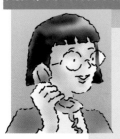

Q: *Today, the physician ordered a throat culture for a six-year-old girl with a sore throat. The patient started to cry. Her mother explained that the little girl hates throat cultures because they make her gag. I did the test as quickly as I could, but what could I have done to reduce the child's anxiety?*

A: It's important to make the experience as positive as possible.
Here are some steps you can take to do this.

1. First, you need to gain the child's trust. Children will follow your instructions more easily if they trust you. Talk *with* your small patient, not *at* her, and don't talk down to her.

2. Next, explain the procedure using words the child can understand. Be honest about any discomfort she may feel. Tell her that when the swab touches the back of her throat, she may gag a little, but that feeling will go away almost immediately. Tell her that if she opens her mouth very wide and says "ahhh" loudly it will make her gag a little less. This gives her a sense of control.

3. Ask if she has any questions and take the time to answer them. If you think it would help, you can give her a swab to hold and touch.

4. As you perform the procedure, open your own mouth wide and say "ahhh" as well. It may help the child to see you doing it.

Regardless of how smoothly the procedure goes, be comforting and reassuring to your patient afterwards.

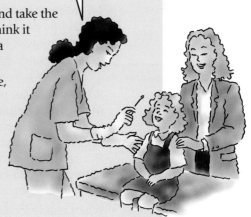

dures are followed. Patients should be told to bring specimens they collect at home to the office or lab as soon as possible.

Most often, the feces is tested for the presence of occult (or hidden) blood. Blood in a patient's stool can mean there's bleeding in the gastrointestinal (GI) tract. This can be a sign of several conditions, including ulcers or colorectal cancer. Other tests may look for ova (eggs) and parasites (O&P). The steps for testing a stool specimen for occult blood can be found in the Hands On procedure on page 247.

TRANSPORTING SPECIMENS

Most pathogens are not fragile. However, every specimen should be processed or transported for processing as soon as possible after it's collected. Otherwise, some organisms in it could multiply or die off. Either event could cause a false result on the test.

Specimens that will be processed in an outside lab must first be placed in transport media. A number of companies manufacture this special type of media. It can generally be stored at room temperature until it's needed for use.

Closer Look   FECAL COLLECTION TIPS

Follow these tips for collecting stool specimens.

- When testing for occult blood, tell the patient to avoid these foods and medications, which can cause false results, for two days before collecting the sample:
  — red meat and fruits high in vitamin C
  — cauliflower, broccoli, lettuce, spinach, corn, and other vegetables that contain the enzyme peroxidase
  — aspirin and nonsteroid anti-inflammatory drugs (NSAIDs)

- When testing for pinworms, collect the sample early in the morning before the patient has a bowel movement or a bath. Pinworms tend to leave the rectum and lay eggs around the anus during the night. Place clear adhesive tape against the anal area. Remove it quickly and place it sticky-side down on a glass slide for the physician or lab to examine.

- When testing for parasites, tell the patient not to use a laxative or enema before the test. This might destroy the evidence of parasites. If the sample contains blood or mucus, include as much of this as possible in the container.

Most transport media are self-contained and include a plastic tube with a sterile swab and media appropriate for transporting that type of specimen. You'll usually find all the directions for using the container on the manufacturer's package.

Fill out all paperwork carefully. Double check the information before releasing specimens for transport. Many specimens that are tested outside the office will be sent to large laboratories. You want to be sure your patient's specimen is identified, processed, and tested properly.

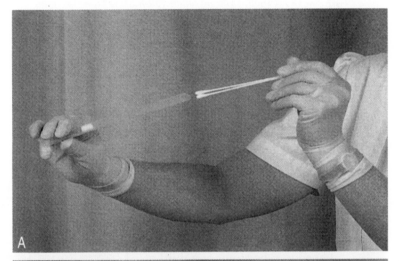

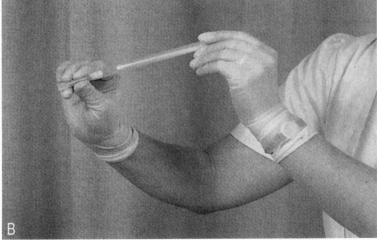

This specimen is being prepared for transport. (A) The swabs are placed in the transport tube. (B) The ampule at the bottom of the tube is squeezed to release the medium into the tube.

For the most reliable results, lab tests should be performed on specimens within an hour after collection. When that isn't possible, store the specimen properly to preserve all its properties. Never expose a specimen to extreme temperature changes. The table on page 233 gives general guidelines for handling common types of specimens.

Running Smoothly

PREPARING A SPECIMEN FOR TRANSPORT

What should you do when you must send a specimen to an outside lab?

It's critical that specimens be prepared quickly and properly for transport. Otherwise, the test results may be worthless. Here are some basic steps to follow when preparing a specimen for transport.

1. Assemble your supplies: the appropriate lab request form, specimen container, and mailing container.

2. Complete the lab request form. Don't leave any questions unanswered.

3. Wash your hands and put on gloves.

4. Check the expiration date and condition of the transport medium.

5. Peel the envelope away from the transport tube about one-third of the way so you can remove the tube.

6. Label the tube with the date, patient's name, source of specimen, and initials of the person processing the specimen.

7. Obtain the specimen as directed by the physician.

8. Return the swab to the tube. Follow manufacturer's instructions for immersion in the medium.

9. Remove and dispose of gloves. Wash your hands.

10. Package for transport as directed on the container. Attach a label to the outside identifying it as a biohazardous biological specimen.

11. Mail the package or contact a courier to pick it up.

> Specimens being sent to outside labs need to be prepared quickly. Before obtaining the specimen, make sure you gather all the necessary supplies and fill out the lab request form.

Handling Common Specimens

Specimen	Collecting	Processing
Urine	Clean-catch midstream with care to avoid contaminating the inside of the container. Don't let stand more than one hour after collection.	Refrigerate if test cannot be performed within one hour.
Blood	Handle carefully. Collect in blood culture bottle. Must remain free of contaminants. Requires special preparation of the venipuncture site.	Deliver to lab immediately.
Feces	Collect in clean container. Leave at room temperature if testing for ova (eggs), parasites, or occult blood.	Deliver to lab at once. If delayed, mix with preservative recommended by lab or use transport medium.
Microbiology specimens	Don't contaminate swab or inside of container by touching either to surface other than site of collection. Protect anaerobic specimens from exposure to air.	Transport as soon as possible.

Culturing Specimens

In medical microbiology, much of the testing to diagnose disease is done using cultures. As you've already read in this chapter, the lab can create the warmth, nutrients, and other things microbes need to grow. There are three types of cultures.

- **Primary cultures** come directly from a patient's specimen. These cultures are used to study any or all of the microorganisms found at the specimen site.

- **Secondary cultures,** also called subcultures, are taken from the primary culture. Suspicious-looking organisms in the primary culture are removed and encouraged to grow for more study.

- **Pure cultures** contain only one type of organism. A pure culture may be either a primary or a secondary culture.

CULTURE MEDIA

You already know that the purpose of media is to encourage the growth of microbes so physicians can identify them easily. When the perfect environment is provided, microorganisms will grow and multiply, making it easier to diagnose and treat a disease.

Whatever the suspected microbe is, all the things it needs to survive must be present for it to grow. The media in the culture container provides nutrients, moisture, and the right pH. The incubator maintains the right temperature and gaseous atmosphere. Depending on the type of suspected microbe, the incubator or the culture containers placed in it provide the correct atmosphere—oxygen for aerobes, no oxygen for anaerobes, or CO_2 for capnophilic organisms.

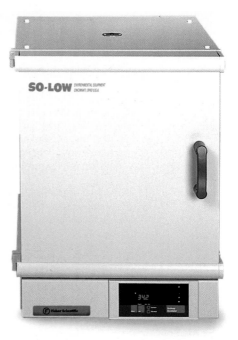

This standard laboratory incubator can be set to provide the right temperature and atmospheric conditions for the bacteria being cultured.

Types of Media

There are three basic preparations, or forms, in which media come:

- solid
- semisolid
- liquid or broth

Media also can be divided into selective and nonselective media.

- **Selective media** contain substances added to the media to help specific organisms grow and to slow the growth of other organisms.
- **Nonselective media** will grow almost any microorganism.

BLOOD AGAR

Most specimens submitted for lab study are cultured on blood agar. This solid medium is prepared by adding five percent sheep's blood to **agar**, a firm, transparent and colorless gelatin-like substance made from seaweed. The agar congeals the blood and forms a firm surface to support the growth of microbes. The firm surface makes it easy to observe the culture growth.

Media Containers

A **petri dish** is an empty glass or plastic container that's used to hold a solid culture medium, such as blood agar. Once the container is filled with the medium, it's called a **plate**. The plate is fitted with a cover to prevent contamination of the specimen. Plates are clear so you can see the culture as it grows.

Agar also may be placed in sterile glass tubes. The tubes are either allowed to harden with a flat-top surface (a butt tube) or with a slanted surface (a slant-and-butt combination).

A liquid or broth medium usually comes in a small jar or tube. Many special broth media have swabs to be used for specimen collection and are enclosed in special envelopes for transporting the specimen.

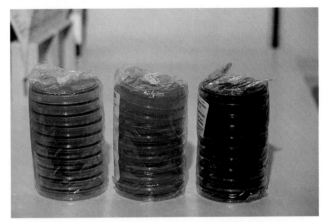

Solid media come on plates wrapped in a plastic sleeve. Plates are always stored medium side up. Plates stored medium side down can develop condensation on the medium, which would interfere with tests.

Caring for Media

Commercially prepared culture media are available for use in medical offices. The media are packaged in disposable plastic plates. Follow these guidelines for preserving the quality and integrity of the plates.

- Date each sleeve when the shipment arrives.
- Store these plates in the refrigerator with the side containing the medium on top. The plates should be stored in the plastic wrapper to keep the medium moist.
- Don't overfill the refrigerator or place media against the back wall or sides. This will raise the temperature.
- Check and record the temperature of the refrigerator daily.
- Rotate the media in the refrigerator so the oldest is in front and is used first. Base the rotation on the date the media expires, not the date it arrived at the office.
- Check the expiration date and the condition of the medium surface before use. Throw away any plates that are past the expiration date and any with media that's dried or cracked.

You should refrigerate the agar until needed. Then warm it to room temperature before use. If the plate is too cold, it will kill many microorganisms.

Most medical offices are equipped with an incubator set at 96 degrees F (35 degrees C). Check and record the incubator temperature daily.

Special Environments

Many labs use special sealed jars or other methods to create a desired gaseous atmosphere. Some special atmospheres are designed for **anaerobic** bacteria (bacteria that live without oxygen). Other special atmospheres are rich in CO_2.

Organisms that grow in increased CO_2 are referred to as **capnophilic.** Capnophilic organisms include strepto-coccus, staphylococcus, *N. gonorrhoeae*, *N. meningi-tidis*, and *H. influenzae.* The environment needed to culture capnophilic microbes can be created in several ways.

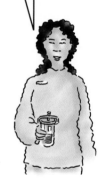

Some organisms, such as capnophilic bacteria, grow best in an environment rich in carbon dioxide.

- Plates can be placed in a sealed jar with a lighted candle. The candle consumes some of the oxygen and produces an atmosphere of five to ten percent CO_2.
- You can add five to ten percent CO_2 to the whole incubator.
- Plates, usually blood agar, are placed in a special sealed jar with an envelope or pouch. You can add water to this pouch to cause a chemical reaction that releases CO_2. This produces an atmosphere of five to ten percent CO_2.

Similar pouches are available that can be used to create anaero-bic conditions.

MICROBIOLOGICAL INOCULATION

Microbiological **inoculation** means introducing a microbe into a culture medium and then putting the medium in an environment likely to make the microbe grow. To make sure a specimen is inoculated in a way that microbes in it will grow best, you'll put it on or in the medium by one of these methods:

- by using a specimen swab
- by removing part of the specimen using a sterile inoculat-ing loop or inoculating needle

The swab and the inoculating loop or needle are used in different situations. Swabs are used when sampling some spec-imens, such as feces, from specimen containers. Other speci-mens, such as sputum, are sampled with loops. A swab is usually used when the specimen is being transferred directly from the patient site onto the culture medium. You would then switch to an inoculating loop to prepare the specimen for culture.

A sterile inoculating loop or needle is used when lifting a colony from a culture to inoculate a secondary culture. Specific colonies are lifted from the primary culture plate and streaked onto the second plate. Then those specific colonies will be incubated again for a pure culture and more study.

Plates

To inoculate a solid medium on a plate, you streak the medium using a qualitative or quantitative technique. Qualitative cultures are done to reveal what kinds of bacteria are present. Quantitative cultures tell how many of a certain bacteria are present. Specific steps for preparing each type can be found in the Hands On procedures on pages 254 and 259.

Butt and Slant Tubes

Butt tubes are inoculated by penetrating the center of the media surface with a needle inoculator, stopping about one-fourth inch from the bottom of the tube.

Slant tubes are usually inoculated with a curvy stroke up the surface of the slant. Some slant tubes require that you inoculate by both streaking the slant and penetrating the center of the butt portion.

Inoculating Other Media

You inoculate a broth or semisolid medium by inserting the swab or loop containing the specimen below the surface of the medium. The illustration on

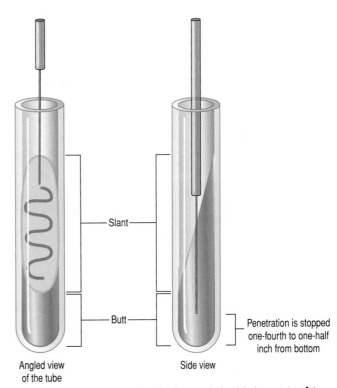

Slant

Butt

Angled view of the tube

Side view

Penetration is stopped one-fourth to one-half inch from bottom

This slant tube requires that you have the slant streaked and the butt portion of the tube penetrated. The penetration is stopped one-fourth to one-half inch from the bottom of the tube.

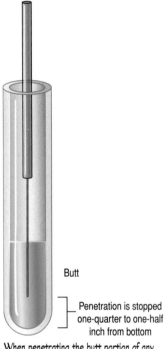

Butt

Penetration is stopped
one-quarter to one-half
inch from bottom

When penetrating the butt portion of any
tube, you should try to enter and remove
the needle through the same line or hole.

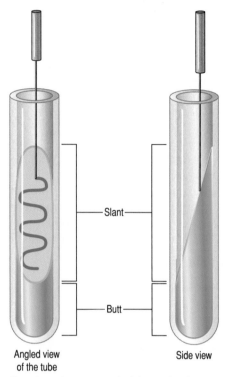

Slant

Butt

Angled view
of the tube

Side view

This culture tube is inoculated only by streaking the slant.

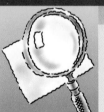

Closer Look

INOCULATING CAPNOPHILIC ORGANISMS

The tubes or bottles used for culturing some capnophilic organisms, such as *N. gonorrhoeae* (responsible for gonorrhea), frequently come with the required carbon dioxide atmosphere already in the container. Be careful to hold the tubes upright while inoculating them. If you tip the tubes, the colorless carbon dioxide gas, which is heavier than oxygen, will pour out—just like water out of a pitcher. If the carbon dioxide is gone, no capnophilic organisms that might be present in a specimen will grow in the culture medium.

this page shows the process for inoculating a liquid medium.

SENSITIVITY TESTING

When the physician wants a specimen cultured, she will usually order what's called a C&S. This stands for *"culture and sensitivity."* It's a several-step test that involves not only growing any pathogens in a specimen, but also finding out which drugs will stop their growth. The physician can then use those drugs to help the patient's body fight off the microbes.

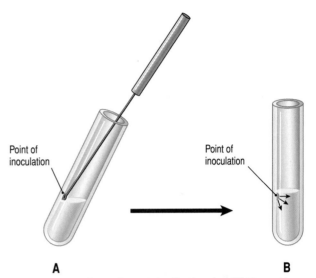

A   **B**

Notice the technique for inoculating a tube of broth medium. (A) Slant and inoculate the side of the tube as shown. (B) Replace the tube upright. This places the point of inoculation below the surface of the medium.

To perform a sensitivity test, a secondary or pure culture of the suspected pathogen is created. A sample from this culture is then inoculated in broth medium and incubated for 18 to 24 hours.

Next, a sterile inoculating loop is used to transfer the growth in this medium into a tube containing another liquid medium. Growth should be added until the second tube is so turbid (cloudy) that print is barely visible through the tube. If not enough growth is available to reach this level of turbidity, the tube can be incubated for two to four hours, until the correct turbidity is achieved.

The contents of the tube are next used to inoculate a culture plate. The Hands On procedure on page 248 will give you the steps for doing this, and for placing disks of various drugs in the medium. The process is also shown in the illustration on page 240.

After the plate is prepared, it's incubated for 18 to 24 hours. It's then inspected to see if there's a zone around any of the disks where no microbes have grown (called a **zone of inhibition**).

- If there's no zone of inhibition around a disk, the pathogen is *resistant* to that particular drug. Therefore, using the drug wouldn't be effective for treating the patient's infection.

- If there's no microbe growth around a disk, you know that the pathogen is *sensitive* to that particular drug. It would be effective for treating the patient.

- If there's a small zone around a disk, this would be reported as an *intermediate* test result. Such a drug would be barely effective against the microbe.

- The best drug to use in treatment will be the one with the largest zone of inhibition. This shows it is the most effective drug against that microbe.

Refer again to the illustration on this page to see how to read a drug sensitivity test.

URINE COLONY COUNTS

Urine cultures often include a colony count in addition to a culture and sensitivity test. A urine colony count measures the amount of bacteria growing in one milliliter of urine. The results can tell the physician the severity of the infection if pathogens are present.

To perform this test, urine is generally inoculated onto two or three types of media. For example, a blood agar plate will grow all bacteria present in the specimen. MacConkey media will grow only gram-negative rods and Columbian CNA media will grow only any gram-positive cocci that may be present. (You'll read about what gram-negative and gram-positive mean shortly.)

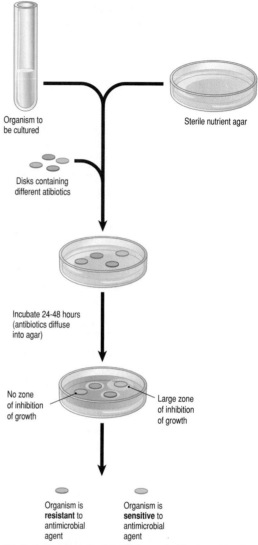

Organism to be cultured

Sterile nutrient agar

Disks containing different atibiotics

Incubate 24-48 hours (antibiotics diffuse into agar)

No zone of inhibition of growth

Large zone of inhibition of growth

Organism is **resistant** to antimicrobial agent

Organism is **sensitive** to antimicrobial agent

This illustration shows the disk diffusion method for determining the sensitivity of bacteria to certain antibiotics.

- 0–100 visible colonies on a plate indicates 0–10,000 bacteria/mL and means that no infection is present.

- 100–1,000 visible colonies on a plate indicates 10,000–100,000 bacteria/mL and means that the patient might have a urinary tract infection (UTI).

- More than 1,000 visible colonies on a plate indicates more than 100,000 bacteria/mL and means that an infection is

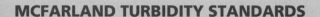

Closer Look   MCFARLAND TURBIDITY STANDARDS

The broth medium used to inoculate a plate in a culture and sensitivity test contains a standard amount of bacteria. The C&S may provide false results if there are too few or too many bacteria present in the broth. To make sure the broth's turbidity is correct before it's inoculated onto the plate, the tube containing it is compared to a known standard called a McFarland standard.

McFarland standards result from mixing sulfuric acid and barium chloride to obtain a solution with a specific turbidity. The most commonly desired turbidity is the McFarland 0.5 standard. This is obtained by mixing 99.5 mL of 1-percent sulfuric acid and 0.5 mL of 1.175-percent barium chloride.

The McFarland tube and the inoculated broth are compared side-by-side against a white card containing several horizontal black lines. The lines must not be easier or more difficult to see through the tube of broth than through the McFarland tube. If the lines can be seen equally well through both tubes, you know that the broth contains the right amount of bacteria for culturing.

Several types of instruments can also measure the McFarland standard of a solution. These machine measurements are generally more accurate than visual comparisons.

definitely present. The higher the number, the more severe the infection is.

As a medical assistant, you probably won't be making these counts. However, you may be asked to inoculate the plates. The Hands On procedure on page 254 gives you step-by-step guidance for inoculating plates for a urine colony count using the "even lawn" streaking technique.

Microscopic Examination

Bacteria grown on a culture can be spread onto a glass slide so they can be examined under a microscope. Sometimes a swab of the specimen is taken directly from the site and put on the slide. Microscopic examination can help identify the specific pathogen that's causing the patient's problems.

LOOKING FOR MICROORGANISMS

Microscopic examination is also used to identify other microorganisms, such as parasites and fungi. For example:

• Stool specimens are put on slides to look for parasites such as pinworms, tapeworms, and their ova.

• Fungi such as "ringworm" and "yeast" infections are diagnosed by examining skin scrapings and samples from mucous membranes under a microscope.

• The protozoa that cause malaria are found through the microscopic examination of blood.

WET MOUNTS AND DRY SMEARS

Some pathogens are easier to identify if they're allowed to move about freely in fluid. This type of slide is called a wet mount. Wet mounts always should be viewed right away, or not later than 30 minutes after the slide is prepared.

You'll find guidance for preparing a wet mount slide in the Hands On procedure on page 263. The Hands On procedure on page 265 will tell you how to prepare a smear—also called a *dry smear*. This is a slide in which the specimen is not suspended in fluid.

Direct smears are slides made from material taken directly from the patient. They may contain epithelial cells (skin cells or cells from organ linings) as well as bacteria or other microbes. Indirect smears are slides made from a culture. They will contain only bacterial cells.

If more than one slide is made from a culture, number the colonies that will be observed on the back of the plate or plates. Then number each slide with the corresponding number using a diamond-tipped pen on the frosted edge of the slide to properly identify its culture site. You may also use a pencil to label the frosted part of the slide.

GRAM STAINING

Most bacteria are colorless. They're hard to identify or even to see without some kind of special treatment. At times, a fixative or a stain is added to the smear. Fixatives are solutions or sprays that "fix" the specimen to the slide. Stains help the physician identify the microbe.

Dutch physician Hans Gram developed the Gram stain process more than 100 years ago. He discovered that after staining with crystal violet and safranin (a red dye), certain bacteria hold the purple color of the crystal violet dye. These bacteria are known as gram-positive bacteria. Other bacteria will stain red with the safranin, which is also called the **counterstain.** These bacteria are called gram negative.

The Gram stain is an important test. Along with factors such as the bacteria's shape and the patient's symptoms, it helps give the physician an idea of the patient's disease. This can allow treatment to begin even before the specimen is cultured. For the steps in Gram staining a smear slide, see the Hands On procedure on page 267.

READING A GRAM STAIN

The Gram stain is read, or interpreted, using a bright-field microscope. The report should include these things:

- the bacteria's morphology (usually cocci or bacilli)
- the bacteria's gram reaction (gram positive if purple or blue, gram negative if red or pink)
- the arrangement of the bacteria (chains or clusters), if there is any significant arrangement

In most medical offices, the physician reads and reports the Gram stain test. However, you will need to observe the slide first to make sure it can be read. If there's a problem, you may have to make and stain a new slide.

Closer Look   STREPTOCOCCAL TESTING

Other methods exist for the rapid detection of certain bacteria. One of these is the rapid strep test.

Strep throat is among the most common infections seen in a physician's office. Because of the need to quickly diagnose and treat this infection, many kits are available to test for this pathogen, group A beta-hemolytic streptococcus (*Streptococcus pyogenes*). The test can be read in just a few minutes. Patients can wait for the results and, if necessary, leave the office with prescriptions in hand.

Rapid strep tests rely on the antigen-antibody reaction, which causes a change on the testing material. (You read about this type of testing in Chapter 4.) Test kit manufacturers provide quick, easy-to-follow instructions. The kits also include quality control measures to let you know if the test is working properly.

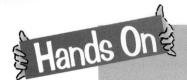

COLLECTING A SPECIMEN FOR THROAT CULTURE

7-1

Follow these steps to collect a specimen for throat culture.

1. Gather your equipment and supplies, including a tongue blade, a sterile specimen container and swab, gloves, a commercial throat culture kit (for testing in your office), a laboratory request form, and a biohazard container (for transport to the lab).

2. Wash your hands and put on gloves.

3. Greet and identify the patient. Explain the procedure.

4. Ask the patient to sit so a light source is directed at his throat.

5. Remove the sterile swab from its container.

6. Ask the patient to say "ahhh" as you press on the midpoint of the tongue with the tongue depressor. Saying "ahhh" helps reduce the gag reflex.

7. Now swab the membranes that are suspected to be infected. Normally, you'll touch the side of the throat at the depth of the tissue hanging in the center back of the mouth (uvula). Expose all of the swab's surfaces to the membranes by turning the swab over the membranes. Avoid touching any other areas with the swab.

8. Keep holding the tongue depressor in place while removing the swab from your patient's mouth.

9. Follow the directions on the specimen container for transferring the swab or processing the specimen in the office.

10. Dispose of supplies and equipment in a biohazard waste container. Remove your gloves and wash your hands.

11. Route the specimen or store it properly until you can route it.

12. Document the procedure.

Charting Example:
11/20/2007 10:30 A.M. Throat specimen obtained as ordered, rapid strep test negative, specimen to Boyton labs for C&S.

_____ M. Mohr, RMA

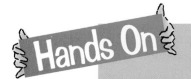

COLLECTING A SPUTUM SPECIMEN

7-2

Follow these steps to collect a sputum specimen.

1. Gather your equipment and supplies, including the labeled sterile specimen container, gloves, the laboratory request form, and a biohazard transport container.

2. Wash your hands and put on gloves.

3. Greet and identify the patient. Explain the procedure. Write the patient's name on a label and put the label on the outside of the container.

4. Ask the patient to cough deeply. Tell the patient to use the abdominal muscles to bring secretions up from the lungs.

5. Ask the patient to expectorate directly into the container. Caution him or her not to touch the inside of the container or the specimen will be contaminated. You'll need 5 to 10 mL for most tests.

6. Handle the specimen container according to standard precautions. Cap the container right away and put it into a transport container marked *biohazard*. Fill out the proper laboratory requisition slip.

7. Care for and dispose of your equipment and supplies. Clean your work area. Then you can remove your gloves and wash your hands.

8. Send the specimen to the laboratory immediately.

9. Document the procedure.

Charting Example:
07/01/2007 12:45 P.M. Moderate amount of thick, yellow sputum obtained and sent to ABC laboratory for a C&S as ordered per Dr. Smith. _____ J. Shapiro, CMA

Hands On

COLLECTING A STOOL SPECIMEN

7-3

Follow these steps in teaching a patient how to collect a stool specimen.

1. Gather your equipment and supplies, including a stool specimen container (for ova and parasite testing), an occult blood test kit (for occult blood testing), and wooden spatulas or tongue blades. Label the container or test kit with the patient's name.

2. Wash your hands.

3. Greet and identify the patient. Explain the procedure. Also explain any dietary, medication, or other restrictions necessary for the collection. (Don't collect a specimen within four days of a barium procedure.)

4. When collecting a specimen for ova and parasites:
   - Tell the patient to collect a small amount of the first and last portion of the stool using the wooden spatula and to place the specimen in the container.
   - Suggest that it's easier if the patient defecates into a disposable plastic container designed to fit on a toilet seat (called a specimen pan, or "top hat") or onto plastic wrap placed over the toilet bowl.
   - Caution the patient not to contaminate the specimen with urine.

5. When collecting a specimen for occult blood:
   - Suggest that the patient obtain the sample from the toilet paper he or she uses to wipe after defecating. Tell the patient to use a wooden spatula to collect the sample.
   - Tell the patient to smear a small amount of the sample from the spatula onto the slide windows.

6. After the patient returns the stool sample, store the specimen as directed. If you're instructing the patient to take the specimen directly to a laboratory, give the patient a completed laboratory requisition form.

7. Document the date and time of the procedure as well as the instructions that were given to the patient, including the routing procedure.

Charting Example:
06/13/2007 3:00 P.M. Pt. given supplies (specimen pack and wooden spatulas) and instructions on obtaining stools for occult blood; instructions on returning slides also given. Pt. verbalized understanding. _____ P. Jones, CMA

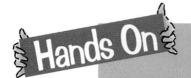

TESTING A STOOL SPECIMEN FOR OCCULT BLOOD   **7-4**

Follow these steps to test a stool specimen for occult blood. This procedure should take five minutes.

1. Gather your equipment and supplies, including gloves, the patient's labeled specimen pack, and developer (or reagent drops). Make sure you check the expiration date on the developing solution. You could get inaccurate test results from expired solution.

2. Wash your hands and put on gloves.

3. Open the test window on the back of the pack. Then put a drop of the developer or testing reagent on each window according to the manufacturer's directions.

4. Read the color change within the time specified by the directions. The time is usually 60 seconds.

5. Put a drop of developer (as directed) on the control monitor section or window of the pack. Take note whether the quality control results are positive or negative, as appropriate.

6. Use proper procedures to dispose of the test pack and gloves. Then wash your hands.

7. Record the procedure.

Charting Example:
03/28/2007 3:00 P.M. Occult blood slides ×3 returned to office via mail; findings positive. Dr. Franklin notified. _____
_____ J. Smith, RMA

Hands On

INOCULATING A CULTURE USING DILUTION STREAKING

7-5

Follow these steps to use dilution streaking to inoculate a medium for a qualitative culture. In a qualitative culture, the physician wants to know if a pathogenic organism is present or not and what the organism is.

1. Gather your equipment and supplies, including the specimen on a swab or loop, gloves, a china marker or permanent lab marker, a sterile or disposable loop, a bacteriological incinerator, and a plate.

2. Wash your hands and put on gloves.

3. Label the medium side of the plate with the patient's name, identification number, source of specimen, your initials, and the date. (The patient's name should be on the side of the plate containing the medium because it's always placed upward to keep moisture from dripping onto the culture.)

4. Use your nondominant hand to remove the media side of the plate from its cover. Then turn it over so the media is toward your face.

5. Using a rolling and sliding motion, streak the specimen swab clear across the top quarter of the plate. Start at the top and work your way to the center. If no additional slides or plates are to be set up on this culture, dispose of the swab in a biohazard container. If the inoculating loop is used for lifting microorganisms for a secondary culture, streak in the same way.

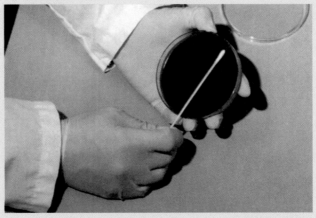

Use a rolling, sliding motion to transfer the specimen to the plate.

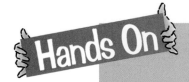

INOCULATING A CULTURE USING DILUTION STREAKING (*continued*)

7-5

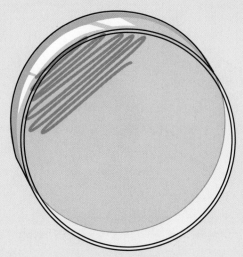

This is the pattern of initial inoculation.

6. If you're inoculating more than one plate using the same sample, perform step 5 on each plate before going on to step 7. Use a new disposable or a sterilized nondisposable loop for each plate.

7.

A. Turn the plate a quarter-turn from its previous position. Pass the loop five to six times through the original streaks and down into the new medium approximately a quarter of the surface of the plate. Then make four to five more streaks without entering the originally streaked area.

B. If you're inoculating a blood agar plate, you'll perform an additional step at this point to show differentiating hemolytic characteristics of the *Streptococcus* species. Two one-half inch long cuts are made one-fourth inch apart in the middle of the second streaking pattern. To do this, turn the loop sideways and cut half the depth of the loop into the media. With the loop halfway in the media, cut approximately one-fourth to one-half inch long. Repeat this step to make a second cut about one-fourth inch

(*continued*)

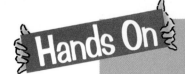

INOCULATING A CULTURE USING DILUTION STREAKING (*continued*)

7-5

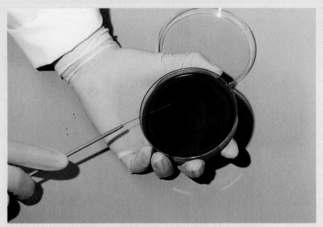

Draw the loop at right angles to the midpoint of the plate.

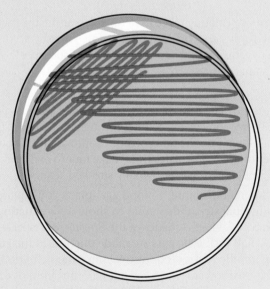

This is the second pattern you'll make.

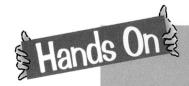

INOCULATING A CULTURE USING DILUTION STREAKING (*continued*)

7-5

away from the first. Hold the loop at a 45-degree angle so the flap of the media closes off the cut and reduces oxygen growth, which is necessary to show the differentiating hemolytic characteristics of *Streptococcus*.

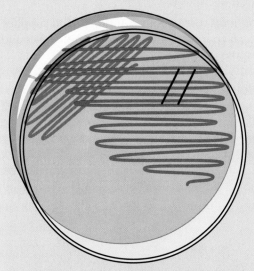

Two additional cuts are made in the second streaking pattern of a blood agar plate. Make sure they're about one-half inch long and about one-fourth inch apart.

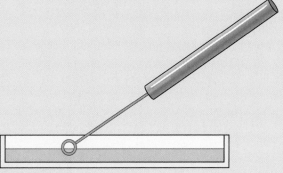

This side view shows what the depth of the loop should be when making the additional cuts in the blood agar plate.

(*continued*)

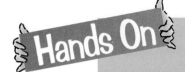

INOCULATING A CULTURE USING DILUTION STREAKING *(continued)*

7-5

8. Turn the plate another quarter-turn so that now it is 180 degrees to the original smear. Working in the same way as in step 7A, draw the loop at right angles through the most recently streaked area 3 to 4 times. Don't enter the original streaked area this time, however.

9. Care for or dispose of your equipment and supplies properly. Clean your work area. Remove your gloves and wash your hands.

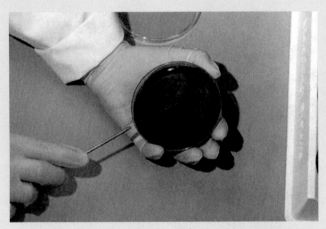

Turn the plate another quarter-turn and streak in the same manner.

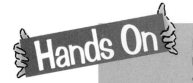

INOCULATING A CULTURE USING DILUTION STREAKING (continued)

7-5

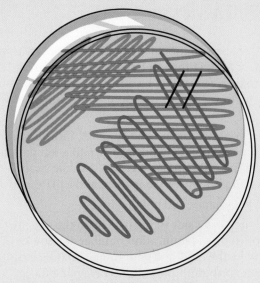

This illustration shows you the complete pattern of specimen inoculation using dilution streaking.

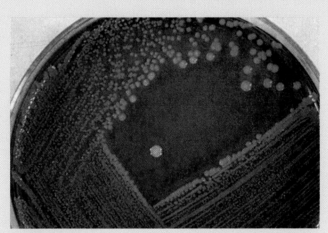

You can clearly see the pale yellow colonies of <u>Staphylococcus aureus</u> on this properly streaked plate.

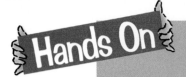

INOCULATING FOR DRUG SENSITIVITY TESTING (KIRBY-BAUER DISK DIFFUSION DRUG SENSITIVITY) USING "EVEN LAWN" STREAKING

Follow these steps to inoculate for drug sensitivity testing (Kirby-Bauer Disk Diffusion Drug Sensitivity) using "even lawn" streaking. Sensitivity testing can be done on 100 mm plates for up to 6 drugs or on 150 mm plates for up to 12 drugs.

1. Gather your equipment and supplies, including a pure broth culture of an organism grown to a standard turbidity (0.5 McFarland standard), gloves, a sterile swab, a china marker or permanent lab marker, and a plate.

2. Wash your hands and put on gloves.

3. Label the media side of the plate with the patient's name and/or culture identification number, the source of the specimen, the date, and your initials. Dating a culture helps to distinguish multiple cultures on a patient.

4. Remove the pure culture tube from the test tube rack. Remove the cap from the pure broth culture. A pure culture is necessary to make sure the sensitivity shows a single organism that's causing the infection.

5. Using your dominant hand, dip the sterile swab into the culture. As you take the swab out of the culture, press and rotate it on the inside of the tube above the level of the broth. This will help remove excess fluid from the swab. Then recap the tube and return it to the rack.

6. Remove the media side of the plate from the cover using your nondominant hand and turn the media toward your face. Remember, the petri dish is always placed on the work surface with the cover down. If you use your nondominant hand for this step, your dominant hand is still free to work with the swab.

7. Starting at one edge of the media, draw the swab down the middle of the plate crossing the diameter of the plate with your streak. Go directly to the next step. Don't change the swab.

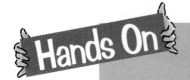

INOCULATING FOR DRUG SENSITIVITY TESTING (KIRBY-BAUER DISK DIFFUSION DRUG SENSITIVITY) USING "EVEN LAWN" STREAKING (*continued*)

7-6

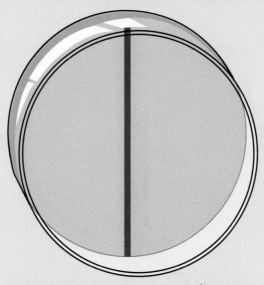

This illustration shows the correct way to draw the first streak on the media with your swab.

8. Using the same swab, streak the plate from side to side at a right angle to the diameter you drew in step 7. Don't leave any space between your streaks in this step.
   - Use this tip—it's easier to start in the middle of the plate and move toward the top edge. Then rotate the plate 180 degrees and streak the other half of the plate, once again starting in the middle.
   - If you don't do a good job spreading the bacteria and you leave space between your streaks, it'll be hard to measure the zones of inhibition in a later step.
   - When you've completed this step, go directly to the next step. Don't change your swab.

9. Now rotate your plate 90 degrees. Streak your plate in the same way you did in step 8. This time, you're streaking parallel to the diameter you drew in step 7. The goal is to

(*continued*)

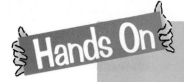

INOCULATING FOR DRUG SENSITIVITY TESTING (KIRBY-BAUER DISK DIFFUSION DRUG SENSITIVITY) USING "EVEN LAWN" STREAKING (*continued*)

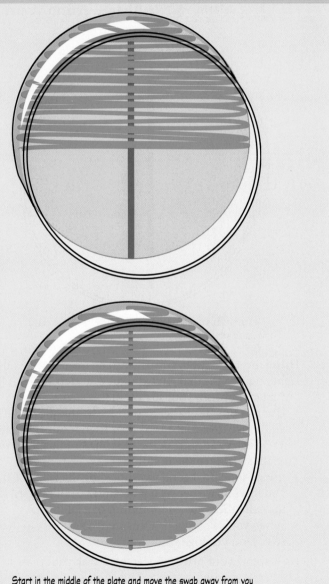

Start in the middle of the plate and move the swab away from you as you streak. That way the rim of the plate won't get in your way.

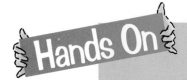

INOCULATING FOR DRUG SENSITIVITY TESTING (KIRBY-BAUER DISK DIFFUSION DRUG SENSITIVITY) USING "EVEN LAWN" STREAKING (*continued*)

spread the bacteria out as much as possible so that when it grows, it will evenly cover every bit of space on the media surface. If you do this step properly, you'll be able to measure the nice round zones of inhibition in a later step.

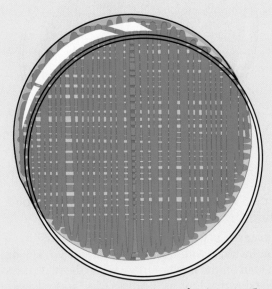

Streak your plate parallel to the diameter you first drew in step 7.

10. Rotate your plate 45 degrees and repeat the streaking using the same method as in steps 8 and 9.

11. Within 15 minutes of completing step 10, you must apply the drug disks to the plate using sterile forceps or an automatic dispenser.
    - Each disk should be pressed down gently using a sterile loop or sterile forceps. Push down until good contact is made with the surface of the agar.
    - Make sure you pay attention to the time limit on this step. Bacteria reproduce about every 20 minutes. If you

(*continued*)

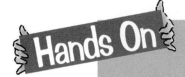

INOCULATING FOR DRUG SENSITIVITY TESTING (KIRBY-BAUER DISK DIFFUSION DRUG SENSITIVITY) USING "EVEN LAWN" STREAKING (*continued*)

7-6

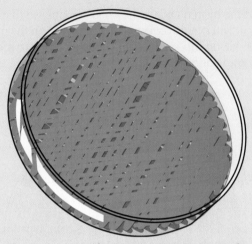

Your streaking in step 10 is diagonal to the streaking in step 9.

wait too long to get the disks on the media, you may get growth where none should exist.

12. Incubate the plates overnight (18 to 24 hours) in an incubator. Incubate with the disk/media side up. The disks won't fall off the media surface when the plate is turned upside down as long as the disks were pressed against the surface of the media.

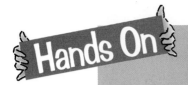

INOCULATING FOR QUANTITATIVE CULTURING OR URINE COLONY COUNT USING "EVEN LAWN" STREAKING

Follow these steps to inoculate plates of media for urine colony counts and for quantitative culturing in general.

1. Gather your equipment and supplies, including a sterile "clean catch" urine specimen, a calibrated .01 mL inoculating loop, a china marker or permanent laboratory marker, and a plate. (Urines are frequently set up on two or three different types of media, for example, blood agar [growth of all organisms], MacConkey [growth of negative rods], or Columbian CNA [growth of positive cocci]. Note the same technique would be used on each plate.)

2. Wash your hands and put on gloves.

3. Label the media side of the plate with the patient's name and/or culture identification number, the source of the specimen, the date, and your initials. Dating the culture helps to distinguish multiple cultures on a patient.

4. Remove the cover from the urine specimen.

5. Using your dominant hand, dip the calibrated loop into the urine specimen. Hold the loop at a right angle (90 degrees) to the surface of the liquid. Withdraw the loop and make sure there's a film of liquid in the loop. If you can't see a film of liquid, repeat this step.

6. Remove the media side of the plate from the cover using your nondominant hand and turn the media toward your face. Remember, the plate is always placed on the work surface with the cover down. If you use your nondominant hand for this step, your dominant hand is still free to work with the inoculating loop.

7. Hold the loop so the flat side of the loop is parallel to the surface of the media. (This will allow the urine to come off the loop and go onto the plate.)
   • Starting at one edge of the media, draw the loop down the middle of the plate, crossing the entire diameter of the plate with your streak.
   • Then go directly to the next step. Don't change loops or sterilize your loop.

(continued)

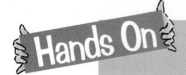
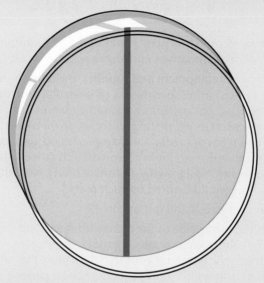

This illustration shows the correct way to draw the first streak on the media with your loop.

8. Using the same loop, now streak the plate from side to side at a right angle to the diameter you drew in step 7. Don't leave any space between your streaks in this step.
   - Here's a tip. It's easier to start in the middle of the plate and move toward the top edge. Then rotate the plate 180 degrees and streak the other half of the plate, once again starting in the middle.
   - Then go directly to the next step. Don't change loops or sterilize your loop.

9. Now rotate your plate 90 degrees. Streak your plate in the same way you did in step 8. This time, you're streaking parallel to the diameter you drew in step 7.

10. Rotate your plate 45 degrees and repeat the streaking using the same method as in steps 8 and 9.

11. Incubate the plate(s) overnight (18 to 24 hours) in an incubator.

12. The visible colonies can be counted the day after incubation and converted to bacteria/mL.

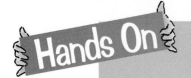
INOCULATING FOR QUANTITATIVE CULTURING OR URINE COLONY COUNT USING "EVEN LAWN" STREAKING (*continued*)

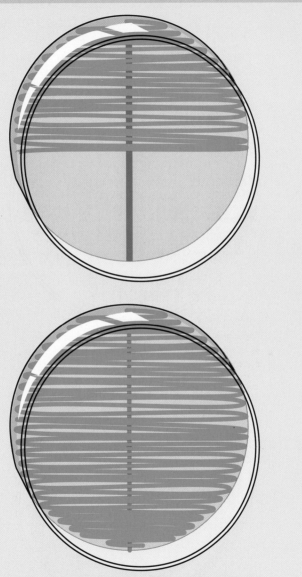

By streaking in this way, you attempt to spread the urine out evenly across the surface of the plate so any bacteria will grow as individual colonies. If they aren't well spread out, they'll grow on top of one another, making it hard to count the number of colonies.

(*continued*)

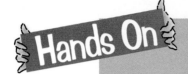

INOCULATING FOR QUANTITATIVE CULTURING OR URINE COLONY COUNT USING "EVEN LAWN" STREAKING (*continued*)

7-7

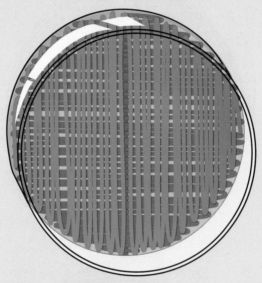

The purpose of streaking this way is to spread the bacteria out as much as you can to make it easier to count the colonies of bacteria later.

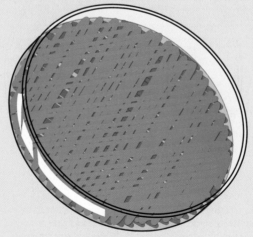

Your streaking in Step 10 is diagonal to the streaking in step 9.

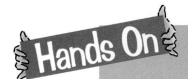

PREPARING A WET MOUNT SLIDE

7-8

Follow these steps to prepare a wet mount slide.

1. Gather your equipment and supplies, including the specimen, gloves, a slide, sterile saline or ten-percent potassium hydroxide (KOH), a coverslip, petroleum jelly, a microscope, and a pencil or diamond-tipped pen.

2. Wash your hands and put on gloves.

3. Label the frosted edge of the slide with the patient's name and the date using a pencil or diamond-tipped pen.

4. Put a drop of the specimen on a glass slide with sterile saline or ten-percent potassium hydroxide (KOH).

5. Use a wooden applicator stick to coat the rim of a coverslip with petroleum jelly.
   - You also can spread a thin layer of petroleum jelly on the heal of your gloved hand, then scrape the edges of the coverslip on it to transfer a thin line to each edge.
   - Change the glove before the next step if you use this method.

6. Put the coverslip over the specimen to keep it from evaporating.

7. Examine the slide with a microscope using the 40-power objective lens with diminished light.

Charting Example:
05/24/2007 9:30 A.M. Specimen taken from right index fingernail bed after removing acrylic and prepared as a KOH wet prep. Fungus detected. Dr. Renke read slide. _____
_____ K. Burns, RMA

(*continued*)

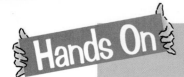

PREPARING A WET MOUNT SLIDE (continued)

7-8

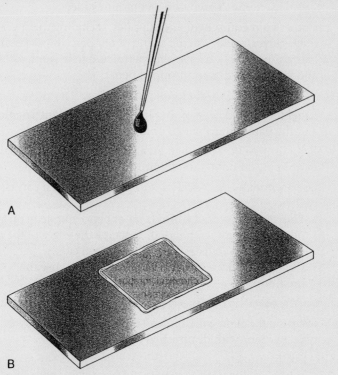

A

B

Here's how to prepare a wet mount slide. (A) Put a drop of the specimen on a glass slide. (B) Ring the edges of a coverslip with petroleum jelly, and then cover the specimen with the coverslip.

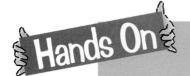

PREPARING A DRY SMEAR

7-9

Follow these steps to prepare a dry smear.

1. Gather your equipment and supplies, including the specimen, gloves, face shield, bacteriological incinerator, slide forceps, slide, sterile swab or inoculating loop, and a pencil or diamond-tipped pen.

2. Wash your hands and put on gloves.

3. Label the frosted edge of the slide with the patient's name and the date using a pencil or diamond-tipped pen.

4. Hold the ends of the slide by the edges between your thumb and index finger.

5. Spread the specimen on the slide using a swab or inoculating loop and start at the right side of the slide.
   - Use a rolling motion with the swab or a sweeping motion with the loop.
   - Spread the material from the specimen gently and evenly over the slide.
   - The material should thinly fill the center of the slide stopping a half inch from each end. You'll avoid contaminating your gloves this way.

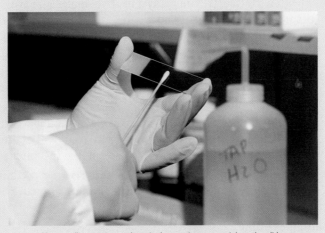

Use a rolling motion to deposit the specimen material on the slide.

(continued)

Hands On

PREPARING A DRY SMEAR (*continued*)

7-9

6. When you're finished placing the specimen on the slide, dispose of the contaminated swab or inoculating loop in a biohazard container. If you're not using a disposable loop, sterilize it using the following steps.
   - Hold the loop in a bacteriological incinerator for five seconds. Don't use a Bunsen burner for this because it may aerosol your specimen. An incinerator confines any aerosol.
   - If you'll be reusing the loop, let it cool so that the heat won't kill the bacteria you'll be putting on it. Don't wave the loop in the air. Waving it around can expose it to contamination. Also, don't stab the medium with a hot loop to cool it off because this will create an aerosol.

7. Allow the smear to air dry in a flat position for at least 30 minutes.
   - Don't wave the slide around in the air or blow on it to speed drying. You could contaminate the specimen with bacteria from your mouth.
   - Don't apply any heat until the specimen has dried. Heat at this point could damage the microorganisms.
   - Some specimens, such as a Pap smear, must be sprayed with a fixative. (If you spray a fixative, make sure you spray four to six inches above the slide.)

8. After drying, hold the dried smear slide with the slide forceps. Then hold the slide in front of the opening of the bacteriological incinerator for eight to ten seconds to "fix" the specimen to the slide. The heat of this process kills the microorganisms and attaches the specimen firmly to the slide.

9. Examine the smear under the microscope or stain it according to your office policy. Usually, the physician will examine the slide to identify the microorganisms in the specimen.

10. Dispose of equipment and supplies in the correct containers. Remove your gloves and dispose of them as well. Then wash your hands.

Charting Example:
07/24/2007 10:00 A.M. Specimen taken from nostril and prepared as direct smear. Gram-positive cocci in chains. Dr. York read the slide. _____ B. White, RMA

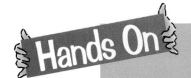

**GRAM STAINING
A SMEAR SLIDE**

7-10

Follow these steps to Gram stain a smear slide. Also note the following precautions:

- Test results may be misinterpreted if a reagent is defective or too near its expiration date.

- Results also may be misinterpreted if you don't closely follow the timing guidelines in the procedure. The bacteria may overstain or color may leach from the cells if time limits aren't observed.

- The results won't be accurate if the specimen wasn't heated properly (to kill the bacteria), if it wasn't incubated long enough, or if the overall dry smear technique wasn't performed correctly.

- To provide better quality control, prepared smears of known gram-positive and gram-negative organisms are processed alongside the patient's specimen when doing this procedure.

1. Gather your equipment and supplies, including crystal violet stain, a staining rack, Gram iodine solution, a wash bottle with distilled water, alcohol-acetone solution, counterstain (for example, safranin), an absorbent (bibulous) paper pad, a specimen on a glass slide labeled with a diamond-tipped pen or a pencil, immersion oil, a microscope, slide forceps, and a stopwatch or timer.

2. Make sure the specimen is heat-fixed to the labeled slide and the slide is at room temperature. See the Hands On procedure on preparing a dry smear on page 265 for guidance.

3. Wash your hands and put on gloves.

4. Put the slide on the staining rack with the smear side up. The staining rack will collect the dye as it runs off the slide.

5. Flood the smear with crystal violet. Then wait for 30 to 60 seconds.

6. Hold the slide with slide forceps and tilt it at a 45-degree angle to drain the excess dye. Then rinse the slide with distilled water for about five seconds and drain off the excess water.

(continued)

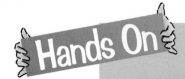

GRAM STAINING
A SMEAR SLIDE (continued)

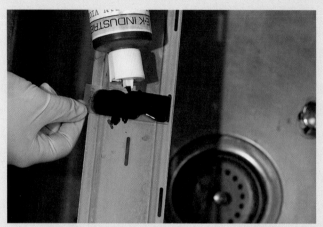

Flood the slide with crystal violet to stain the bacteria purple.

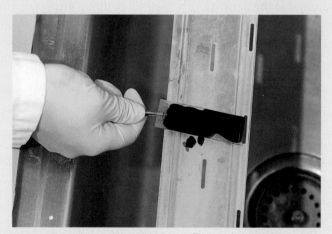

Tilt the slide so the excess dye runs off into the staining rack.

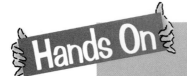

GRAM STAINING
A SMEAR SLIDE (*continued*)

7-10

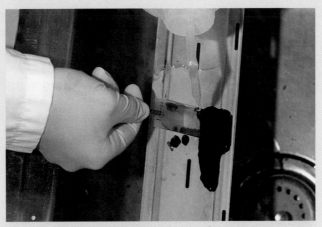

Rinse the slide with water to stop the coloring process.

7. Put the slide back on the slide rack. Now flood the slide with Gram iodine solution and wait 30 to 60 seconds. The iodine will "fix" the crystal violet to the gram-positive bacteria.

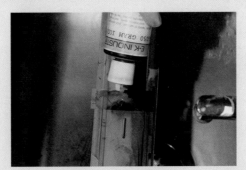

Flood with Gram iodine solution.

8. Using the slide forceps, hold the slide at a 45-degree angle to drain the iodine solution. While the slide is tilted, rinse the slide with distilled water from the wash bottle for five to ten seconds. Then slowly and gently wash the slide with the

(*continued*)

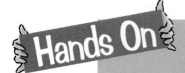

**GRAM STAINING
A SMEAR SLIDE (continued)**

7-10

alcohol-acetone solution for about five to ten seconds, until no more stain runs off. The alcohol-acetone removes the crystal violet stain from the gram-negative bacteria, but the gram-positive bacteria will keep the purple dye.

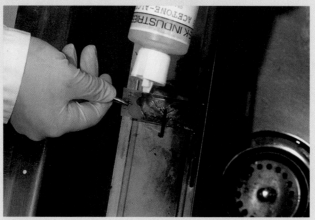

Rinse with alcohol-acetone solution until no more purple stain runs off, about five to ten seconds.

9. Immediately rinse the slide with distilled water for five to ten seconds and return it to the rack. The rinsing will stop the decolorizing process.

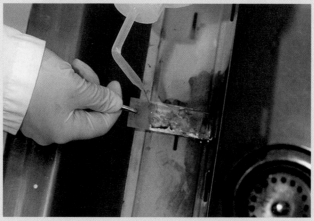

Use distilled water to rinse off the alcohol-acetone solution.

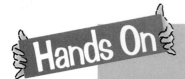

**GRAM STAINING
A SMEAR SLIDE (continued)**

7-10

10. Now, flood the slide with safranin or other appropriate counterstain. Then time a 30- to 60-second wait. The gram-negative bacteria will stain pink or red with the counterstain.

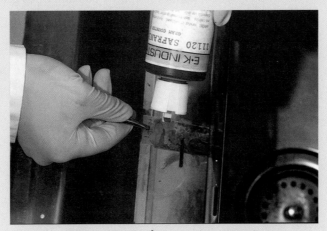

Flood the slide with safranin or another counterstain.

11. Drain the excess counterstain by tilting the slide at a 45-degree angle. After draining the counterstain, rinse the slide with distilled water for five to ten seconds to remove what remains.

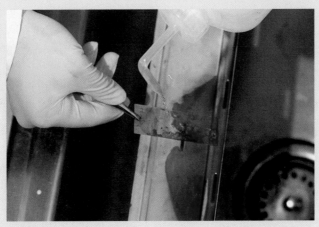

Rinse with distilled water for five to ten seconds to remove the counterstain.

(continued)

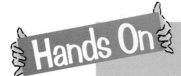

**GRAM STAINING
A SMEAR SLIDE (*continued*)**

7-10

12. Gently blot the smear dry with bibulous paper. Be very careful not to disturb the smeared specimen. Wipe off any solution on the back of the slide. You can put the slide between the pages of a bibulous paper pad and press gently to remove any moisture.

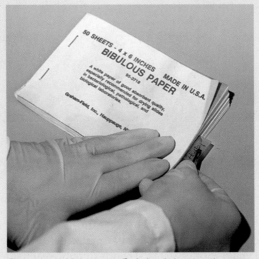

Blot gently with bibulous paper. Don't disturb the smeared specimen.

13. Inspect the slide using the oil immersion objective lens. Remember that you are inspecting only for proper preparation. The physician is the one who interprets the slide.

14. Care for or dispose of your equipment and supplies properly. Clean your work area. Remove your gloves and wash your hands.

Charting Example:
08/14/2007 11:30 A.M. Specimen taken from sputum and Gram stained on a smear slide. Gram-positive cocci in chains. Dr. Barton read the slide. _____ A. Crosby, RMA

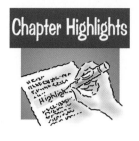

Chapter Highlights

- Microbiology is an important part of the practice of medicine. Your duties in this area may include collecting, processing, and routing specimens, and assisting the physician or patient with specimen collection.

- Commonly collected specimens for microbiological testing include blood, urine, sputum, feces, wound drainage, and mucus. Collection methods include the use of swabs, venipuncture, centesis, and collecting body excretions.

- The major types of microorganisms that you may deal with in your work as a medical assistant include bacteria, viruses, fungi, protozoa (one-celled parasites), and metazoa (parasitic worms and arthropods).

- Follow procedures carefully to avoid contaminating specimens you collect. Also, know how to maintain the quality of each specimen before it is tested. Follow all handling guidelines in dealing with specimens that will be sent to outside labs for processing.

- Bacterial cultures are one way to identify pathogens that may be causing a patient's health problems. This type of testing involves inoculating various kinds of media with specimen samples and then incubating the culture to encourage the pathogens to grow.

- Microscopic examination is another way of identifying bacteria and some fungi and protozoa that cause disease. Wet mounts, dry smears, and Gram staining are all procedures that aid in this process. It's important that you know how to prepare these slide specimens.

GLOSSARY

acidosis   a condition of excess acid in the body fluids [Chapter 6]

aerobic   requiring oxygen to live; contrast with *anaerobic* [Chapter 7]

aerosol   a gas or air that has tiny particles suspended in it [Chapter 1]

agar   a type of seaweed or algae that helps solidify culture media; the media may be referred to as agar [Chapter 7]

agglutination   the clumping together of particles, red blood cells, or bacteria, usually in response to the presence of antibodies [Chapter 4]

alkalosis   a condition of excess base (alkali) in the body fluids [Chapter 6]

ammonia   a substance produced by decomposition of organic matter containing nitrogen [Chapter 5]

amylase   excretory enzyme released by the exocrine system into the intestines to aid in digestion [Chapter 6]

anaerobic   able to live without oxygen; contrast with *aerobic* [Chapter 7]

anemia   deficiency in hemoglobin or in the numbers of red blood cells [Chapter 3]

anion   a negatively charged ion (an atom or group of atoms that has an electrical charge); contrast with *cation* [Chapter 6]

anisocytosis   blood abnormality in which red blood cells are not equal in size [Chapter 3]

antecubital space   inner surface of the bend of the elbow where the major veins for venipuncture are located [Chapter 2]

antibodies   complex globulins produced by B lymphocytes in response to an antigen; molecules that the body identifies as non-self [Chapter 4]

anticoagulant   anything that prevents or delays the clotting of blood [Chapter 1]

antigen   protein markers on cells that cause formation of antibodies and react specifically with those antibodies [Chapter 4]

antiseptic   any substance that inhibits the growth of bacteria; used on skin before any procedure that breaks the integumentary barrier [Chapter 2]

atherosclerosis   buildup of fatty plaque on the interior lining of arteries causing the arteries to narrow and harden [Chapter 6]

autoimmune disease   a disease caused by a person producing antibodies against his or her own cells or tissue [Chapter 4]

bacilli   rod-shaped or cylindrical organisms [Chapter 7]

bacteriology   the science and study of bacteria [Chapter 7]

bevel   slanted cut at the end of a needle that allows the needle to penetrate the vein easily; prevents coring (removal of a portion of skin or vein) [Chapter 2]

bicarbonate   the dissolved form of carbon dioxide; it combines with water to make carbonic acid; carbonic acid loses one of its hydrogen ions to then form bicarbonate [Chapter 6]

bile   a bitter, yellow-green secretion of the liver stored by the gallbladder; derived from bilirubin, cholesterol, and other substances; emulsifies fats in the small intestine so they can be further digested and absorbed [Chapter 6]

bloodborne pathogens   viruses that can be spread through direct contact with blood or body fluids from an infected person [Chapter 1]

buffy coat   the middle layer of a blood specimen containing white blood cells and platelets that forms when blood has been centrifuged [Chapter 1]

calibration   part of the process of setting calculation points for a lab instrument by processing solutions of known values within the instrument's reportable range; necessary for maintaining quality control of lab instruments [Chapter 1]

capillary   a very fine and slender blood vessel [Chapter 2]

capnophilic   requiring an atmosphere that is high in carbon dioxide to live [Chapter 7]

cation   a positively charged ion (an atom or group of atoms that has an electrical charge); contrast with *anion* [Chapter 6]

centesis   surgical puncture made into a cavity [Chapter 7]

centrifugal force   a spinning motion to exert force outward; heavier components of a solution are spun downward [Chapter 1]

centrifuge   machine that uses centrifugal force, or spinning to exert force outward, to separate blood and other fluids into their component parts [Chapter 1]

chlamydiae   parasitic microorganisms with properties common to bacteria but unable to sustain life without a host, in the manner of a virus [Chapter 7]

Clinical Laboratory Improvement Amendments (CLIA) guidelines established by Congress in 1988 to standardize and improve laboratory testing [Chapter 1]

cocci bacteria that are spherical in form [Chapter 7]

colony a group of bacteria or cells growing on a solid nutrient surface [Chapter 7]

counterstain stain used to color parts of a microscopy specimen that are not affected by the primary stain [Chapter 7]

creatine a chemical compound in the body that adds phosphorus to ADP (adenosine diphosphate) to make ATP (adenosine triphosphate), which is the energy currency of the body [Chapter 6]

culture a laboratory process whereby microorganisms are grown in a special medium, often for the purpose of identifying a causative agent in an infectious disease [Chapter 7]

differential diagnosis a systematic way of determining which of two or more diseases with similar symptoms a patient is suffering from [Chapter 6]

diuretics medications that increase the production of urine in the body [Chapter 5]

donor a person who contributes blood [Chapter 4]

edema an accumulation of fluid within the tissues that causes swelling [Chapter 6]

elliptocytosis a condition in which all or almost all of the red blood cells are elliptical or oval in shape; typically asymptomatic [Chapter 3]

endocrine system the body system that consists of the endocrine glands (such as the pituitary, thyroid, and adrenal glands) and the hormones they secrete [Chapter 6]

enzyme a protein that begins (catalyzes) a chemical reaction [Chapter 3]

erythrocytes red blood cells [Chapter 3]

erythropoietin a hormone produced mainly by the kidneys in response to lowered oxygen levels; stimulates the production of red blood cells to increase blood oxygen levels [Chapter 3]

esterase an enzyme that splits esters (compounds similar to salts) [Chapter 5]

exocrine system sweat glands and other glands that release their secretions directly to the body's cavities, organs, or surface through a duct [Chapter 6]

external control tested in the same manner as a patient's sample; however, its value or expected result is already known [Chapter 4]

extracellular fluid all the body fluids that exist outside the cells, including the blood and fluid in spaces between tissue cells (interstitial fluid), constituting about 20 percent of the body's weight [Chapter 6]

false-negative a test result that fails to detect the substance being tested for, even though it is present in the specimen [Chapter 4]

false-positive a test result that says a substance is present in a specimen when it actually is not [Chapter 4]

femtoliter one quadrillionth of a liter [Chapter 3]

flagella hair-like extremities of a bacterium or protozoan that are used to facilitate movement [Chapter 7]

folate a salt of folic acid; it acts to help enzymes that build structures such as blood cells [Chapter 3]

galactosuria condition in newborns lacking an enzyme that metabolizes galactose; increased levels of galactose appear in the blood and urine (if proper therapy is not initiated, mental retardation and other difficulties will occur) [Chapter 5]

gauge diameter of a needle lumen [Chapter 2]

gestational diabetes a disorder characterized by an impaired ability to metabolize carbohydrates, usually due to insulin deficiency occurring in pregnancy and usually disappearing after delivery [Chapter 6]

glucagon hormone that stimulates the release of glycogen when blood glucose levels drop [Chapter 6]

glycogen the stored form of glucose, found mainly in the muscles and liver [Chapter 6]

glycosuria the presence of glucose in the urine [Chapter 5]

gout a disorder in the body's metabolism of uric acid, marked by high levels of uric acid in the blood, and deposits of urate crystals in and around the joints, leading to arthritis and painful inflammation of the joints, especially in the hands and feet [Chapter 6]

graduated something that is marked at intervals (as in a container) in order to allow the measurement of its contents [Chapter 1]

hematocytometer device for counting blood cells (also known as *hemocytometer*) [Chapter 3]

hematology study of blood and blood-forming tissues and diseases of the blood [Chapter 3]

hematoma blood clot that forms at an injury site [Chapter 2]

hematopoiesis blood cell production [Chapter 3]

hematuria blood in the urine [Chapter 5]

hemoconcentration a condition in which the plasma portion of the blood filters into the tissues, causing an increase in nonfilterable blood components, such as red blood cells, enzymes, iron, and calcium [Chapter 2]

hemocytometer   device for counting blood cells (also known as *hematocytometer*) [Chapter 3]

hemoglobin   an iron protein pigment found in red blood cells that carries oxygen and carbon dioxide in the blood stream [Chapter 3]

hemoglobin C disease   an inherited anemia marked by an excessive destruction of red blood cells, an enlarged spleen, target cells (a type of red blood cell), and abnormal hemoglobin (called hemoglobin C) in the blood [Chapter 3]

hemolysis   rupture of red blood cells with the release of hemoglobin into the plasma or serum causing the specimen to appear pink or red in color [Chapter 2]

hemolytic anemia   a disorder characterized by premature destruction of the red cells; this may be brought on by an infectious process, inherited red cell disorders, or as a response to certain drugs or toxins [Chapter 3]

hemostasis   process by which the body stops the leakage of blood from the vascular system [Chapter 3]

hyperglycemia   an increase in blood sugar, as in diabetes mellitus [Chapter 5]

hyperosmolarity   a condition of having increased numbers of dissolved substances in the plasma [Chapter 3]

hypoxia   a condition characterized by insufficient levels of oxygen in the blood and tissues [Chapter 3]

immunohematology   the testing performed by blood banks on red blood cells and serum or plasma to study the antigen-antibody reaction including the study of autoimmunity [Chapter 4]

inoculation   introduction of a weakened form of a pathogen (such as a bacteria or toxic agent) into the body to stimulate the body to produce antibodies and thus create immunity to the condition or disease [Chapter 7]

internal controls   tools built into a serology test kit to ensure that test procedures are followed correctly and that reagents are working properly [Chapter 4]

intracellular fluid   the liquid contained within a tissue's cells [Chapter 6]

intravascular coagulation   clot formulation within the vessels; strands of fibrin may form from one wall of the vessel to the other and shear red cells as they pass by [Chapter 3]

ions   an atom or group of atoms that has become electrically charged by the loss or gain of one or more electrons [Chapter 6]

isoenzyme   a term applied to any enzyme in a group of enzymes that have a similar function in the body but different physical and chemical properties [Chapter 6]

leukemia   an increase in white blood cells characterized by the presence of a large number of abnormal forms [Chapter 3]

leukocytes   white blood cells [Chapter 3]

lipase   any of several enzymes that begin the breakdown of fats in the digestive tract [Chapter 6]

lipemic   having an excess of fat in the blood [Chapter 4]

lipids   any of the free fatty acids in the body [Chapter 6]

lipoprotein   a substance made up of a lipid and a protein [Chapter 6]

Luer adapter   a device for connecting a syringe or evacuated holder to the needle to promote a secure fit [Chapter 2]

lymphocyte   a nongranular leukocyte; a type of white blood cell (WBC) that helps the body develop immunity; normally, between 22 and 28 percent of WBCs are lymphocytes [Chapter 3]

lyse   to cause disintegration (i.e., destruction of adhesions, or the breakdown of red blood cells) [Chapter 5]

Material Safety Data Sheet (MSDS)   required written information about a hazardous substance kept at a site, including instructions on how to use it safely, precautions for preventing accidents or injuries, and first aid and other measures to take if an accident or injury occurs [Chapter 1]

media   special material used when culturing specimens that helps bacteria present in the specimen to grow [Chapter 7]; **selective media** may contain additives to support the growth of specific organisms and inhibit the growth of others [Chapter 5]

megaloblastic anemia   a disorder characterized by the production of large, dysfunctional erythrocytes; folate deficiency is considered a cause [Chapter 3]

microbe   a commonly used but nontechnical synonym for *microorganism* [Chapter 1]

microorganisms   living organisms that can be seen only with the aid of a microscope [Chapter 1]

monocyte   a large white blood cell that surrounds and absorbs microorganisms and other foreign bodies in the blood and tissues; normally, between three and eight percent of a person's WBCs are monocytes [Chapter 3]

morphology   a description of the physical characteristics and form and structure of an organism, including bacteria and red blood cells [Chapter 3]

mycology   the science and study of fungi [Chapter 7]

myelofibrosis   a disorder in which bone marrow tissue develops in abnormal sites such as the liver and spleen; signs include immature cells in the circulation, anemia, and splenomegaly [Chapter 3]

neutrophil a type of white blood cell that is highly destructive of microorganisms; the most common type of white blood cell in the body [Chapter 3]

nitrogenous pertaining to or containing nitrogen, usually the end product of protein metabolism [Chapter 6]

nitroprusside a nitrogen cyanic compound that reacts with ketones [Chapter 5]

nonselective media culture media in which many different types of bacteria can grow [Chapter 7]

normal flora microorganisms normally found in the body that do not cause disease; also known as resident flora [Chapter 7]

normal values acceptable range as established for an age, a population, or a sex; variations usually indicate a disorder [Chapter 1]

nosocomial infections infections acquired in a medical setting, generally presumed to be in a hospital setting but may also refer to a medical office [Chapter 7]

obligate to require; a parasite that has no choice but to attach to a living organism [Chapter 7]

opportunistic relating to an organism that is capable of causing disease in a host only when the host's resistance is low [Chapter 7]

palpate to examine by feeling and pressing with the palms and fingers [Chapter 2]

parasitology the science and study of parasites [Chapter 7]

particulate matter tiny solid particles [Chapter 5]

pathogens disease-causing microorganisms [Chapter 7]

peripheral blood the volume of blood circulating in the body [Chapter 3]

petri dish a shallow glass or plastic dish with a lid to hold solid media for cultures [Chapter 7]

phlebotomist medical professional who draws blood from patients [Chapter 1]

phlebotomy the procedure for withdrawing blood from the body [Chapter 2]

phosphate a compound containing phosphorus and oxygen; very important in living organisms, especially for the transfer of genetic information [Chapter 5]

picogram a measure of weight that is one trillionth of a gram; abbreviated *pg* [Chapter 3]

plasma the clear, fluid part of the blood in which the blood's cells are suspended; contrast with *serum* [Chapter 1]

plate a dish-like container that contains a thin layer of culture media [Chapter 7]

poikilocytosis abnormal variations in the shapes of red blood cells (poikilo = variation) [Chapter 3]

precipitation the settling out of a substance in a solution [Chapter 5]

primary culture comes directly from the patient's specimen and is used to investigate any or all of the microorganisms found at the specimen sight [Chapter 7]

prophylaxis protective treatment for the prevention of disease once exposure has occurred [Chapter 2]

pure culture a culture that contains the growth of only one kind of bacteria and that is free of any other microorganisms [Chapter 7]

quality assurance (QA) an evaluation of health care services as compared to accepted standards [Chapter 1]

quality control (QC) method to evaluate the proper performance of testing procedures, supplies, or equipment in a laboratory [Chapter 1]

quality control specimens samples that have the values that cover the calibrated range of a lab instrument; necessary for maintaining quality control of lab instruments [Chapter 1]

reagent a substance used to react in a certain manner in the presence of specific chemicals to obtain a diagnosis [Chapter 1]

reportable range range in which analyzers, procedures, or instruments are designed to produce results [Chapter 1]

Rh factor any of several substances on the surface of red blood cells that produce a strong antibody response in individuals whose blood lacks the substance, if both kinds of blood come into contact through pregnancy or transfusion [Chapter 4]

rickettsias parasitic microorganisms with properties common to bacteria but unable to sustain life without a host, in the manner of a virus; cause Rocky Mountain spotted fever, typhus, Q fever, and trench fever and carried by a certain kind of tick, louse, or mite [Chapter 7]

saline a solution of sodium chloride in sterile water that is commonly used in IV infusions and in irrigating some parts of the body (such as nasal passages) [Chapter 4]

secondary culture suspicious organisms taken from the primary culture and encouraged to grow for more extensive study; also called subcultures [Chapter 7]

sediment solid matter suspended in a liquid that sinks to the bottom through settling or after the liquid has been centrifuged [Chapter 5]

selective media   culture media in which only certain types of bacteria will grow [Chapter 7]

sensitivity   susceptibility to a certain substance [Chapter 4]

serology   the study of the nature and properties of different types of body fluids [Chapter 4]

serum   the fluid that remains after fibrinogen and other clotting factors have been removed from blood plasma; contrast with *plasma* [Chapter 1]

sickle cell anemia   a condition in which the patient has both copies of the gene for hemoglobin S; the red cells become sickle shaped and nonflexible causing obstruction of small vessels and capillaries; necrosis due to tissue hypoxia occurs beyond the obstruction; most commonly seen in African Americans [Chapter 3]

skin puncture   procedure requiring penetration of the capillary bed in the dermis of the skin with a lancet or other sharp device [Chapter 2]

specificity   design of antibody to recognize and bind with only one kind of antigen [Chapter 4]

specimen   a small portion of anything used to evaluate the nature of the whole [Chapter 1]

spectrophotometer   an instrument that measures light in a solution to determine the concentration of substances in it [Chapter 6]

spherocytosis   a condition where all or almost all of the red cells are spherocytes; typically asymptomatic [Chapter 3]

spirochete   a long, flexible, motile microorganism [Chapter 7]

spore   bacterial life form that resists destruction by heat, drying, or chemicals; spore-producing bacteria include botulism and tetanus [Chapter 7]

staphylococci   spherical microorganisms found on all surfaces of the skin and on many mucous membranes; some can cause skin infections [Chapter 7]

streptococci   spherical bacteria that may cause sore throat, scarlet fever, rheumatic fever, many pneumonias, and various skin infections [Chapter 7]

supernatant   the liquid that remains after a fluid is centrifuged [Chapter 5]

syncope   sudden fall in blood pressure or cerebral hypoxia resulting in loss of consciousness [Chapter 2]

thalassemia   a hemolytic anemia caused by deficient hemoglobin synthesis; more commonly found in those of Mediterranean heritage [Chapter 3]

thrombocytes   platelets [Chapter 3]

thromboplastin   a complex substance found in blood and tissues that aids the clotting process [Chapter 3]

titer   measure of the amount of an antibody in serum [Chapter 4]

turbid   the condition of a liquid being cloudy [Chapter 5]

urates   nitrogenous compounds derived from protein use that are excreted in the urine [Chapter 5]

vacuum   a space from which air has been removed [Chapter 2]

vein   any of the blood vessels that carry unaerated blood from the tissues toward the heart [Chapter 2]

venipuncture   the puncture of a vein in order to withdraw blood, infuse IV fluids, or administer medicines [Chapter 2]

virology   the science and study of viruses [Chapter 7]

whole blood   blood from which none of its component parts (for example, plasma or platelets) has been removed [Chapter 3]

zone of inhibition   the area around an antibiotic on a culture plate, in which no bacteria have grown [Chapter 7]

FIGURE CREDITS

Illustrations in *Medical Assisting Made Incredibly Easy: Lab Competencies* have been borrowed from the following sources:

Bayer Corporation, Elkhart, IN (chapter 5, unnumbered figures 15–17).

Bayer HealthCare LLC, Diagnostics Division, Tarrytown, NY (chapter 5, unnumbered figures 5, 10–13).

Beckman-Coulter, Fullerton, CA (chapter 3, unnumbered figure 4).

Becton-Dickinson, Franklin Lakes, NJ (chapter 2, unnumbered figures 5, 10A, 10C, 11A, and 12; chapter 3, unnumbered figure 6).

Cholestech, Heywood, CA (chapter 6, unnumbered figure 14).

Cohen BJ, Taylor J. Memmler's Structure and Function of the Human Body. 8th ed. Baltimore: Lippincott Williams & Wilkins, 2005 (chapter 3, unnumbered figure 1).

Cohen BJ. Memmler's The Human Body in Health and Disease. 10th ed. Baltimore: Lippincott Williams & Wilkins, 2005 (chapter 4, unnumbered figure 13).

Cygnus Inc, Redwood City, CA (chapter 6, unnumbered figure 8).

Evans-Smith P. Taylor's Clinical Nursing Skills: A Nursing Process Approach. Philadelphia: Lippincott Williams & Wilkins, 2005 (chapter 2, unnumbered figure 16; chapter 6, unnumbered figures 15–18).

Goodheart HP. Goodheart's Photoguide of Common Skin Disorders. 2nd ed. Philadelphia: Lippincott Williams & Wilkins, 2003 (chapter 7, unnumbered figure 7).

Greiner Bio-One, Kremsmuenster, Austria (chapter 2, unnumbered figure 11B).

ITC, Edison, NJ (chapter 2, unnumbered figures 10B and 10D; chapter 3, unnumbered figure 11).

McCall RE, Tankersley CM. Phlebotomy Essentials. 3rd ed. Baltimore: Lippincott Williams & Wilkins, 2003 (chapter 1, unnumbered figures 6 and 11; chapter 2, unnumbered figures 9, 17, 19, and 23–31; chapter 5, unnumbered figure 3; chapter 6, unnumbered figures 11 and 13).

Molle EA, Kronenberger J, Durham LS, West-Stack C. Lippincott Williams & Wilkins' Comprehensive Medical Assisting. 2nd ed. Baltimore: Lippincott Williams & Wilkins, 2005 (chapter 1, unnumbered figures 2, 8, 9, 15, and 18; chapter 2, unnumbered figures 1 and 4; chapter 3, unnumbered figures 3 and 13–21; chapter 7, unnumbered figures 3, 11, 14, 19A, 20-32, 34, 38, and 40).

Nikon, Melville, NY (chapter 1, unnumbered figure 4).

Quidel, San Diego, CA (chapter 4, unnumbered figures 9 and 11).

So-Low Environmental Equipment, Cincinnati, OH (chapter 7, unnumbered figure 13).

Ulster Scientific, Highland, NY (chapter 3, unnumbered figure 9).

INDEX

Page numbers in *italics* denote figures; those followed by a t denote tables.

A

ABO blood groups, 126–127, 126t, *129*, 129–130, 130t
ACETEST, 149, 152, 172, *173*
Acid citrate dextrose (ACD), 42t
Acidosis, 188
Addison's disease, 207t
Additives, for blood samples, 40–45, 41t–44t
Aerosol safety, 81–82
Agar media, 234–236, *235*
Agglutination tests, 114–115, 119
    for blood typing, *129*, 129–130, 130t
AIDS (*see* HIV disease)
Alanine aminotransferase (ALT), 192, 193
Albumin, 193
Alcohol abuse, 188, 190 (*see also* Substance abuse)
Alkaline phosphatase (ALP), 192, 193
Alkalosis, 188
American Red Cross, 131–132
Ammonia, in urine, 149–150
Ammonium crystals, *160*
Amylase, 195–196
Anaphylaxis, 112
Anemia, 77, 87
    hemolytic, 88, 128
    megaloblastic, 88t–89t
    tests for, 89
Angina, 205
Anions, 185
Anisocytosis, 88
Antecubital space, 52, *53*
Anthrax, 221
Antibodies, 111–115
Anticoagulants, 6, 40, 95

B

Antigens, 111
    tests for, 113–115
    types of, 127–128
Antiseptics, 36
Arrhythmias, 186
Arthritis, 90, 114, 121
Aspartate aminotransferase (AST), 192, 193
Aspirations, 8
Atherosclerosis, 203–205, 207t
Athlete's foot, 222
Autoclave, 221
Automated cell counter, 16–17
Autopsies, 8

B

Bacilli, *219*, 220, 221
Bacteria, 217–221, *219*
    anaerobic, 236
    capnophilic, 236, 238
    colonies of, 217, 240–241
    spores of, 220, 221
Basophils, 75, *76*, 85, 87t
Bicarbonate (HCO$_3$), 188
Bile, 190, 203
Bilirubin, 146t, 176–177, *177*
    production of, 191–192
    tests for, 149, 153–154
Biohazards, 18–19, *20*
    containers for, *4*, 24, 25
    disposal of, 202, *203*, 216–217
Biopsies, 8
Bladder catheterization, 138
Bleeding time test, 95–96
Blood culturing, 65–68, *66–69*, 233–237, 233t
Blood drawing (*see* Phlebotomy)
Blood glucose test, 27t
Blood typing, 113, 125–132, 126t, *129*, 130t
Blood urea nitrogen (BUN), 189, 207t

Bloodborne Pathogens Standard, 21–22
Body fluid exposure, 63–64
Borrelia burgdorferi, 225
Botulism, 220, 221
Breast-feeding, 111
Broth culture media, 237–239, *239*
Buffy coat, *13*, 113
Burr cells, 89t
Butt tubes, *237–238*
Butterfly set, 46, *47*, *48*

C

Calcium, 187, 207t
Calcium oxalate crystals, 158, *160*
Calibration, 30–31
Cancer, 78, 124
Candidiasis, *160*, 161, 222
Capnophilic organisms, 236, 238
Carbohydrate metabolism, 78, 151–152, 195–196
Cardiac function tests, 194–195
Cardiac risk calculation, 205, 206t
Casts, urinary, 158, *159*
Catheterization, bladder, 138
Cations, 185
Centers for Medicare and Medicaid Services (CMS), 26–29, 33
    scope of practice and, 27t, 79, 190, 226
    Website of, 27
Centesis, 227
Centrifuge, 13–14, 155, 179
Certified medical technologist, 9t
Cestodes, 223–224
Chain of custody (COC), 10
Chemistry analyzers, 14
Children
    abuse of, 141
    needle gauges for, 37–38
    newborn screening of, 48–50, *51*
    skin puncture for, 46–50, *49*, *50*
    throat culture for, 229
    urine specimen from, 139–141
Chlamydiae, 220–221
Chloride, 186–187, 207t
Cholesterol, 27t, *203*, 203–205, 206t, 207t
Clean-catch method, 137–138, 145, 158, 164–165, 233t
CLIA (*see* Clinical Laboratory Improvement Amendments)
Clinical chemistry, 6–7, 182–212

cardiac function and, 193–195
liver function and, 190–193
normal values for, 183, 207t
pancreatic function and, 195–206
renal function and, 184–190
scope of, 182–184
thyroid function and, 193
Clinical Laboratory Improvement Amendments (CLIA), 26–28, 27t, 33
    scope of practice and, 27t, 79, 190, 226
    urinalysis and, 137, 155, 156, 169, 172
    Website of, 27
Clinitest, 149–152, 169–170, *171*
Clostridium spp., 221
CMS (*see* Centers for Medicare and Medicaid Services)
Coagulation tests, 27t, 79, 92–96, *94*
    additives for, 41t–44t
Cocci, 218–220, *219*
Complete blood count, 79–92, *80*, *82*, 86t–89t, *90*
Confidentiality, 7, 84, 123, 163, 206
Containers
    biohazard, *4*, 24, 25
    microcollection, 47
    sharps, 24, 36, 63, 202, *203*
    specimen, *231*, 232, 233t
Coumadin, 6, 94, 95
Creatine, 189
Creatine kinase, 194–195
Creatinine, 189, 207t
Crystal violet stain, 242–243
Crystals, urinary, 158, *159*, *160*, 190
Culture and sensitivity (C&S) testing, 239–240, *240*, 254–258, *255–258*
Culturing, 27t, 215–217, 224–226, 233t
    of blood, 65–68, *66–69*
    Gram staining and, 242–243, 267–272, *268–272*
    inoculation for, 236–239, *237–239*, *248–262*
    media for, 217, 218, 233–239, *234*, *235*, *239*, *240*
    quantitative, 237, *248–253*
    specimens for, 217, 226–230
    types of, 233
    of urine, 27t, 138, 143–145, 240–241
Cushing's syndrome, 185, 207t

Custody, chain of, 10
Cystine crystals, *160*
Cytogenetics, 8, 27t
Cytologist, 9t
Cytology, 8

D

D antigen, 127, 130
Decontamination procedures, 216
Dehydration, 147–148, 207t
Diabetes insipidus, 147, 185, 207t
Diabetes mellitus, 5, 148, 150, 207t
  gestational, 200
  tests for, 27t, 143, 150–152,
    197–200
Diazo tablet test, 149, 154, 176–177,
  177
Dilution streaking technique, *248–253*
Dipstick, urine, 142–143, *144*,
  166–167
Disseminated intravascular coagula-
  tion (DIC), 89t
Diuretics, 146
Draw, order of, 58, 59t
Drugs (*see* Substance abuse)
Drug sensitivity testing, 239–240,
  240, 254–258, *255–258*
Dry smears, 242, *265*, 265–272,
  268–272
Duffy antigen, 128
Dysentery, 223

E

Ear infections, 220
Eclampsia, 207t
Edema, 184
EDTA (*see* Ethylenediaminetetraacetic
  acid)
Ehrlich units, 154
Electrolytes, 185–188
ELISA (*see* Enzyme-linked
  immunosorbent assays)
Elliptocytosis, 89t
Endocrine system, 194
Entamoeba spp., 223
Enzyme-linked immunosorbent
  assays (ELISA), 115–117, 119, 162
Eosinophils, 75, *76*, 85, 86t
Epithelial cells, in urine, *157*,
  158–161
Epstein-Barr virus (EBV), 121
Erythrocytes (*see* Red blood cells)

Erythrocyte sedimentation rate (ESR),
  27t, 79, *90*, 90–91, *106–108*
Erythropoietin, 87–88
Esterase, 154
Ethylenediaminetetraacetic acid
  (EDTA), 69t, 80, 104, 204
Evacuated tube system, 37–40, 41t–44t
"Even lawn" streaking technique, 241,
  254–260, *255–262*
Exocrine system, 195
Extracellular fluid, 185
Eyewash station, 24–25, *25*

F

Fainting, 56
False test results, 114–116, 121, 123,
  167
Fasting blood sugar (FBS), 197–198,
  211
Feces (*see* Stool specimen)
Fibroids, 124
Filter paper test, 48–50, *51*
Finger stick, *70*, 70–72, 80, 104
Flagella, 220
Flammability, *20*
Flora, normal, 215, 222
Flukes, 223–224
Fluorescent treponemal antibody-
  absorption (FTA-ABS) test, 122
Folate deficiency, 84, 88, 89t, 90
Food and Drug Administration
  (FDA), 26–29, 162
Fungi, 221–222, 242

G

Galactosuria, 150–151
Gallbladder, 191, 203
Gangrene, gas, 220, 221
Gas chromatography/mass spectrom-
  etry (GC/MS), 162
Gestational diabetes, 200
Giardia spp., 223
Glassware, 14–15, *15*
Gloves, 22, 26, 27, 36, 216
Glucagon, 196
Glucose tests
  blood, 27t, 150, 197–201, *208–210*
  meters for, *197*, 201, *208–210*
  normal values for, 197, 207t
  urine, 143, 150–152, 212
Glucose tolerance test (GTT),
  198–199, *200*, 211–212

Glycogen, 196
Gonorrhea, 236, 238
Gout, 189–190, 207t
Gram staining, 242–243, 267–272,
268–272
Granular casts, 159
Granulocytes, 75, 76

H

Haemophilus influenzae, 236
Hazardous Communication
(HazCom) Standard, 22
HCG (*see* Human chorionic
gonadotropin)
Heart attack, 195, 205
Heart failure, 185
Heel puncture, 48–50, 49–51, 70–72,
71, 72
Heel warmers, 50
Helminths, 223–224
Hematocrit test, 14, 79, 89
Hematology, 6, 74–109
blood components and, 75–77, 76
coagulation tests and, 92–96, 94
complete blood count and, 79–92,
80, 82, 86t–89t, 90
Hematoma, prevention of, 61
Hematopoiesis, 77
Hematuria, 146, 152, 153
Hemoconcentration, 53, 54
Hemocytometer, 80
Hemoglobin, 75, 88t
blood donors and, 131
tests for, 27t, 79, 81, 91, 199–200
Hemoglobin C disease, 89t
Hemolysis, 38, 116, 156
Hemolytic anemia, 88, 128
Hemostasis, 77
Heparin, 94
for blood samples, 41t–44t, 59t, 204
monitoring of, 6
Hepatitis
biohazards and, 19
chemical, 193
immunization for, 21
needlestick injuries and, 62–63
tests for, 121, 153
Herpes, 223
High-density lipoprotein (HDL), 205,
206t
Hippuric acid crystals, 160
Histocompatibility, 27t
Histology, 8, 9t

HIV disease, 19
antiviral drugs for, 223
needlestick injuries and, 62–63
patient privacy and, 7, 84
Human chorionic gonadotropin
(HCG), 123, 132–133, 161–162
Human immunodeficiency virus (*see*
HIV disease)
Human leukocyte antigens (HLA), 128
Hyaline casts, 159
Hypercalcemia, 187
Hyperchloremia, 187
Hyperchromasia, 88t
Hyperglycemia, 150, 208
Hyperkalemia, 186
Hypernatremia, 185
Hyperosmolarity, 89t
Hyperparathyroidism, 207t
Hyperphosphatemia, 188
Hyperthyroidism, 194, 207t
Hyperuricemia, 189
Hypocalcemia, 187, 188, 207t
Hypochloremia, 187
Hypochromasia, 88t
Hypoglycemia, 198–199, 208
Hypokalemia, 186
Hyponatremia, 185
Hypoparathyroidism, 187, 188, 207t
Hypophosphatemia, 187–188
Hypothyroidism, 194, 207t
filter paper test for, 48–50
hyponatremia from, 185
Hypoxia, 88

I

Ictotest, 149, 154, 176–177, 177
Immunity
disorders of, 78, 121
types of, 111–112
Immunoglobins (Ig), 111, 112
Immunohematology, 7, 113,
125–132, 129, 130t
Immunology, 7, 110–112
reagents for, 117–121
tests for, 113–117, 121–125
Incident reports, 25–26
Incubators, 15, 218, 234, 236
Infants (*see* Children)
Influenza, 27t, 236
Inhibition, zone of, 239–240, 240
Inoculation, 236–239, 237–239,
248–262
Insect bites, 224

Insulin, 186, 196
intracellular fluid, 186
Ions, 182, 185
Iron deficiency, 88t–89t, 90
Isoenzymes, 194–195

K

Kell antigen, 128
Ketoacidosis, 186
Ketones, urine test for, 149, 152
Kidd antigen, 128
Kidney disease, 207t
    hypokalemia from, 186
    renal failure from, 185–188, 207t
    urine pH in, 150
    urine tests for, 152–153, 174–175
Kidney stones, 153, 158, 207t
Kirby-Bauer Disk Diffusion (*see* Drug
    sensitivity testing)
"Kissing disease" (*see* Mononucleosis)
Kova system, 166

L

Laboratories, 10–17, 30–31 (*see also*
    Safety)
    false test results from, 114–116, 121,
        123, 167
    glassware for, 14–15, *15*
    inspection of, 28–29
    regulation of, 26–28, 27t
    staff of, 8, 9t, 33
    standards for, 3, 28–33
    types of, 3–8
Laboratory assistant, 9t
Lancets, 47
Legal issues
    with chain of custody, 10
    with confidentiality, 7, 84, 123,
        163, 206
    with consent, 54
    with drug testing, 10, 163
    with OSHA violations, 22
    with scope of practice, 27t, 79, 190,
        226
Leucine crystals, *160*
Leukemia, 77, 207t
Leukocytes (*see* White blood cells)
Leukocyte esterase, 154–155
Leukopenia, 83
Lewis antigen, 128
Lipase, 195–196
Lipids, 201–204
Lipoproteins, 201–205, *203*, 206t

Liver enzymes, 192
Liver failure, 207t
Liver flukes, 224
Liver function tests, 190–193
Low-density lipoprotein (LDL),
    204–205
Luer adapter, 46, *47*
Lupus erythematosus, 121
Lyme disease, 220, 225
Lymphocytes, 75, *76*, 85, 86t
Lymphogranuloma venereum, 221

M

Macrocytosis, 89t, 90
Magnesium, 187
Malaria, 223, 242
Material safety data sheets (MSDS),
    17–18, 22
McFarland standard, 241
Mean cell volume, 89
Mean corpuscular hemoglobin
    (MCH), 81, 91
Mean corpuscular hemoglobin con-
    centration (MCHC), 91
Mean corpuscular volume, 89–90
Measurement units, 78t
Media, culture, 217, 218, 233–239,
    234, 235, 239, 240
Medical laboratory technician, 9t
Megaloblastic anemia, 88t–89t
Meniscus, *16*
Metabolic disorders, 78, 151–152,
    186–187, 195–196
Metazoa, 223–224
Meters, glucose, *197, 208–210*
Metric prefixes, 78t
Microbiology, 7–8, 215–272 (*see also*
    Microscopy)
    culturing for, 233–241, *234–240*
    specimens for, 224–232, *231*, 233t
    techniques of, 241–272, *248–265,*
        268–272
Microcollection equipment (*see* Skin
    puncture)
Microcytosis, 89t, 90
Microhemagglutination assay (MHA),
    122
Microhematocrits, 14, 27t, 47, *50,*
    104–105, *105*
Microscopy, *11*, 11–12 (*see also*
    Microbiology)
    provider-performed, 27–28, 156
    for urine sediment, 155–161,
        157–160

MNS antigen, 128
Monocytes, 75, *76*, 85, 87t
Mononucleosis, 85, 114, 121–122
MSDS (material safety data sheets), 17–18, 22
Multiple myeloma, 152, 207t
Muscular dystrophy, 207t
Mycology, 222
Myelofibrosis, 89t
Myocardial infarction, 195, 205

N

National Fire Protection Association (NFPA), 19, *20*
Needles
    disposal of, 24, 36, 63, 202, *203*
    gauges of, 37–38
    injuries from, 38, 62–63
    positioning of, 56–57, *57*
    safety features for, 38, *40*
Neisseria gonorrhoeae, 236, 238
Neisseria meningitidis, 236
Nematodes, 223–224
Neoplastic disorders, 78, 124
Nephrolithiasis, 153, 158, 207t
Neutropenia, 84
Neutrophilia, 84
Neutrophilic band, 86t
Neutrophils, 75, *76*, 83–84, 86t
Nitrite test, 154, 158
Nitrogenous compounds, 188–190
Nitroprusside reaction, 152, 172, *173*
Normal flora, 215, 222
Normal values, 183, 207t
Nosocomial infections, 215–217
Nutritional disorder(s), 78, 152, 207t
    gout as, 189–190
    vitamin deficiencies as, 84, 88, 89t, 90

O

Occupational Safety and Health Administration (OSHA), 19–22, 38 (*see also* Safety)
Opportunistic infections, 222
Order of draw, 58, 59t
Otitis media, 220

P

Pancreatic function tests, 195–206
Pancreatitis, 196, 207t

Papanicolaou (Pap) test, 8, 27t
Parasites
    arthropod, 224
    helminthic, 223–224
    obligate, 221, 223
    stool specimen for, 230, 242
Partial thromboplastin time (PTT), 94–95
Pathogens, 215
Pathologist, 9t
Pathology, 8
Peripheral blood smear, 82, 100–102, *101*
Pertussis, 220
Petechiae, 93
Petri dishes, 234–236, *235*, 254
Phenazopyridine, 146t, 167, 176
Phenylketonuria (PKU) test, 48–50, *51*
Phlebotomists, 3, 9t
Phlebotomy, 35–72
    complications from, 58–62, 60t
    equipment for, 36–50, *39*, *40*, 41t–44t, *45–50*
    fainting from, 56
    order of draw for, 58, 59t
    procedures for, 50–58, *53*, *55*, *57*, 65–72, *66–72*
    site selection for, 54–56
Phosphates, 146
Phosphorus, 187–188, 207t
Pinworms, 224, 230, 242
PKU (phenylketonuria) test, 48–50, *50*
Plasma, *13*, 131
Plasmodium spp., 223
Platelets, *13*, 75, *76*, 113
    injections of, 131
    tests for, 91–92
Pneumonia, 220
Poikilocytosis, 88
Postprandial glucose test, 198
Potassium, 186, 207t
Practice, scope of, 27t, 79, 190, 226
Prefixes, metric, 78t
Pregnancy
    diabetes during, 200
    patient privacy and, 7
    proteinuria from, 152
    tests for, 27t, 123–124, 132–133, 161–162
Privacy, 7, 84, 123, 163, 206
Protein, urine test for, 149, 152–153, 174–175
Prothrombin time (PT), 79, 94

Protozoa, 223, 242
Provider-performed microscopy (PPM), 27–28, 156
PTT (partial thromboplastin time), 94–95
Pyridium (*see* Phenazopyridine)
Pyrvinium pamoate, 146t
Pyuria, 152 (*see also* Urinary tract infections)

Q

Q fever, 221
Quality assurance (QA) program, 2–3, 29–33
Quality control (QC)
    external controls for, 118–119
    for reagents, 29–30, 118
    for test kits, 118, 120
    for urinalysis, 155, 156, 169, 172
    logs for, 17–18, 22, 30

R

Rabies, 112
Radioactive substances, 19, 20
Rapid plasma reagin (RPR), 122–123
Reagents, 2, 114, 117–118
    for blood types, 130t
    quality control of, 29–30, 118
    storing of, 117
    for urinalysis, 142–143, 144, 148–149, 149t, 166–167
Red blood cells, 13, 75, 76, 113 (*see also* Blood typing)
    abnormalities of, 88t–89t
    complete cell count of, 87–91, 88t–89t, 90
    storage of, 131
    in urine, 155–156, 157, 159
Refractometer, 148
Refrigerators, 16, 17
Renal failure, 185–188, 207t (*see also* Kidney disease)
Renal function tests, 184–190
Rh factor, 127, 130–131
Rheumatic fever, 218
Rheumatoid arthritis, 90, 114, 121
RhoGAM, 111–112, 127, 128
Rickettsias, 220–221
"Right to know" law (*see* Hazardous Communication Standard)
Ringworm, 222, 242
Rocky Mountain spotted fever, 221

Roundworms, 223–224
RPR (rapid plasma reagin), 122–123
Rubella, 114

S

Safety, 17–26, 202 (*see also* Biohazards; Occupational Safety and Health Administration)
    with aerosols, 81–82
    with Clinitest, 151, 152
    with fainting patient, 56
    with nosocomial infections, 216–217
    with radioactivity, 19, 20
    with sharps, 24, 36, 38, 40, 63, 202, 203
Safranin, 242–243
Salmonellosis, 220
Scarlet fever, 218
Schistocytes, 89t
Schistosomiasis, 224
Scope of practice, 27t, 79, 190, 226
"Sed rate" (*see* Erythrocyte sedimentation rate)
Sediment, urine, 155–161, 157–160, 178–179
Sensitivity, specificity versus, 114
Sensitivity testing, 239–240, 240, 254–258, 255–258
Serology (*see* Immunology)
Serum, 13
Sexually transmitted diseases (STDs), 7, 220–221 (*see also* HIV disease)
    gonorrhea and, 236, 238
    reporting of, 123
    syphilis and, 84, 114, 122–123, 219, 220
Sharps, 24, 36, 38, 40, 63, 202, 203
Sickle cell disease, 89t, 156
Skin puncture
    complications with, 60t, 62
    equipment for, 46–50, 49, 50
    procedure for, 58, 70–72
Slant tubes, 237–238
Sodium, 185, 207t
Sodium polyanethole sulfonate, 42t
Specificity, sensitivity versus, 114
Specimens, 226–227
    blood, 65–68, 66–69, 233t
    collecting of, 5
    containers for, 24, 25, 231
    culture, 217, 226–230
    processing of, 9t
    quality control of, 29–31

Specimens (*continued*)
  sputum, 228, 245
  stool, 228–230, 242, 246–247
  transport of, *4*, 230–232, *231*, 233t
  urine, 137–140, 143–145, 233t
Spectrophotometer, 183, 184
Spherocytosis, 88t, 89t
Spills and splatters, 23–25, 63–64
Spirochetes, *219*, 220
Spores, bacteria, 220, 221
Sputum specimen, 228, 245
Squamous cells, *157*
Staining
  Gram, 242–243, 267–272, *268–272*
  of peripheral blood smear, 102
Staphylococcal infections, *219*, 220,
    236, *253*
Stool specimen, 228–230, 233t,
    246–247
Streaking technique
  dilution, *248–253*
  "even lawn," 241, 254–260,
    255–262
Streptococcal infections, 218–220, *219*
  culturing of, 236
  tests for, 114, 124–125, *125*,
    133–134, 227–229, 243, 244
Substance abuse
  patient privacy and, 7
  tests for, 10, 162–163
  withdrawal syndromes and, 188
Sulfonamides, 146t
Sulfosalicylic acid test, 149, 152–153,
    174–175
Supernatant urine, 155
Suprapubic aspiration, 138–139
Syncope, 56
Syphilis, 84, 220
  cause of, 122, *219*
  reporting of, 123
  tests for, 114, 122
Syringes, *45*, 45–46
  needle gauges and, 37–38
  plunger of, 46
Systemic lupus erythematosus (SLE),
    121

T

Tapeworms, 223–224, 242
Target cells, 89t
Testicular tumor, 124
Tetanus, 220, 221
Thalassemia, 88t–89t

Thixotropic gel, 45
Throat cultures, 27t, 114, 124–125,
    125, 133–134, 227–229, 243, 244
Thrombocytes (*see* Platelets)
Thrombocytopenia, 93
Thrombocytosis, 92
Thyroid function test, 194
Thyroxine (T$_4$), 194
Tinea, 222
Tourniquet, 37, 52–54, *55*
Toxoplasma spp., 223
Trachoma, 221
Transplants, 128
Trematodes, 223–224
Trench fever, 221
Treponema pallidum, 122, *219* (*see also*
    Syphilis)
Trichinosis, 224
Trichomoniasis, *160*, 161, 223
Triglycerides, *203*, 204, 206, 207t
Triiodothyronine (T$_3$), 194
Triple phosphate crystals, 158, *160*
Troponin, 195
Tuberculosis, 19, 84, 220
24-hour urine collection, *140*,
    140–142
Two-hour postprandial glucose test,
    198
Typhus, 221
Tyrosine crystals, *160*

U

Unopette system, *96–99*
Urates, 146
Urea, 189
Uric acid, 189
  crystals of, 158, *159*, *160*, 190
  normal values for, 207t
Urinalysis, 8, 27t, 137–179
  collecting specimens of, 137–140,
    143, 233t
  confirmation tests of, 149
  drug testing by, 10, 162–163
  pregnancy testing and, 161–162
  reagent strips for, 142–143, *144*
  24-hour, *140*, 140–142
Urinary tract infections (UTIs)
  colony counters for, 240–241
  hematuria from, 153
  proteinuria from, 152
  tests for, 153–156, 158
  trichomoniasis and, 223
  urine pH in, 150

Urine
   casts in, 158, *159*
   chemical properties of, 148–155,
      149t
   collecting specimens of, 137–140,
      143
   crystals in, 158, *159*, *160*, 190
   cultures of, 27t, 138, 143–145,
      240–241
   pH of, 149–150, 149t
   physical properties of, 140–142,
      145–148, 145t, 146t, 168
   random, 137
   sediment in, 155–161, *157–160*,
      178–179
   specific gravity of, 145t, 147–148
   supernatant, 155
Urinometer, 148
Urobilinogen, 154
Urobilirubin, 192
UTIs (*see* Urinary tract infections)

V

Vaccination, 111
Vaginitis, 223
Vegetarianism, 150
Venipuncture (*see* Phlebotomy)

Vibrio spp., *219*, 220
Virology, 223
Viruses, 223
Vitamin deficiencies, 84, 88, 89t, 90

W

Warming devices, 50
Westergren test, *90*, 90–92, *106–108*
Wet mounts, 242, 263, *264*
White blood cells, *13*, 75, *76*, 113
   complete blood count of, 80–83
   differential of, 103
   immunoglobin and, 112
   normal values for, 82
   in urine sediment, 156, *157*, *159*
   UTIs and, 154–155
Whooping cough, 220
Winged infusion set, 46, *47*, *48*

Y

Yeast, *160*, 161, 222, 242

Z

Zone of inhibition, 239–240, *240*